MARIA AHLGREN

BEAUTY
FOOD

85 recipes for
health & beauty
from within

PHOTOGRAPHY
LINA EIDENBERG ADAMO

MITCHELL
BEAZLEY

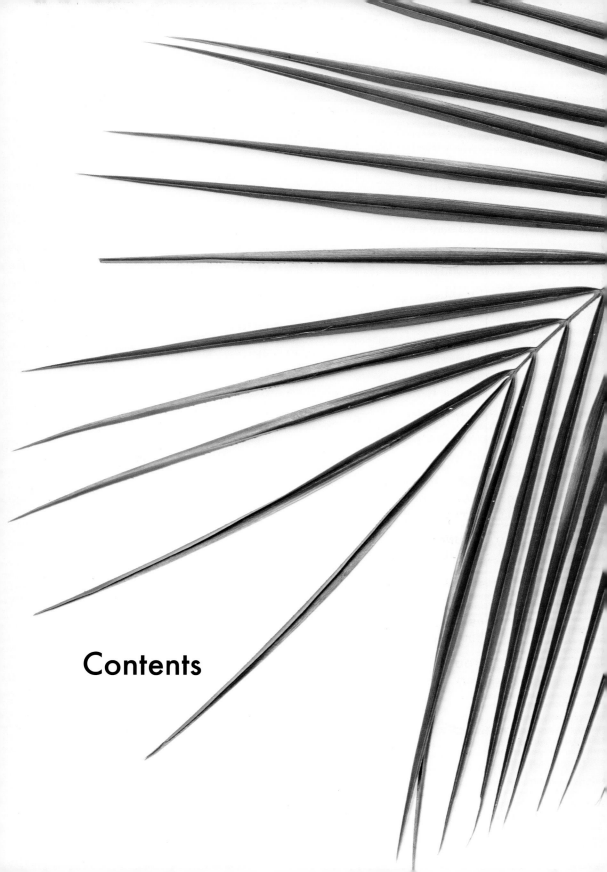

Contents

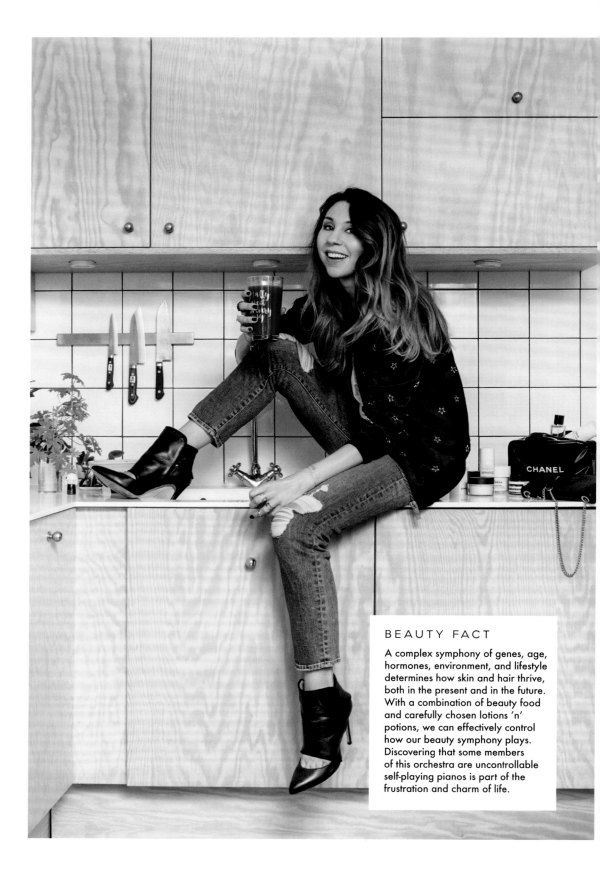

BEAUTY FACT

A complex symphony of genes, age, hormones, environment, and lifestyle determines how skin and hair thrive, both in the present and in the future. With a combination of beauty food and carefully chosen lotions 'n' potions, we can effectively control how our beauty symphony plays. Discovering that some members of this orchestra are uncontrollable self-playing pianos is part of the frustration and charm of life.

Hi there, glow lover!

My name is Maria and I'm obsessed with skincare. Pursuit of the "Great Glow" is my ongoing project, and has been since I was a teenager and dipped my finger in my mother's Lancôme jar for the first time. For more than ten years, I have written for glossy magazines about beauty, and I am currently a beauty editor at Sweden's largest fashion magazine.

A humble brag: I'm a little over 35 and I still get asked for ID to buy alcohol. For that, I thank my parents, my outrageously privileged bathroom cabinet, and my kitchen pantry. In the kitchen, you can create beauty magic—and I'm not just talking about crushed banana face masks or hair treatments made from eggs (although eggs are currently one of the trendiest ingredients in Korean skincare). No, it's all about the food that provides your skin and hair with the best defense against life's trials.

As much as I love silky creams with miraculous promises, high-tech serums, and Cinderella-masks that erase everything from clogged pores to traces of sleepless nights (I'm hopeless when it comes to sleeping), I love to fuel my insides with food that gives my skin the strength to tackle beauty's saboteurs (more about them on page 18).

I spend at least as many hours in the kitchen as in the bathroom. Beauty food is devilishly delicious and easy to make without losing your mind. In this book, I offer several of my favorite recipes to take you through mornings, quick lunches, tasty dinners, television marathons, evening parties, and cozy brunches.

Before we dive into the recipes, I want to emphasize one thing. The skin is the body's biggest organ and a window display of what's happening inside. Like the rest of the body, the skin has two ages—the chronological (the date in our passport) and the biological. The latter is what we see in the mirror.

The skin's condition is a combination of age, genetic inheritance, hormones, and lifestyle. We cannot change our birthdate or parents, but with a combo of beauty food and good skincare, we can take control of the skin's—and hair's—longevity and give them all the conditions necessary to sail through life in peak condition. Everyday beauty saboteurs don't have a chance if we mobilize on all fronts. Fascinating new research in epigenetics has even shown that it is possible to outsmart certain things that are written in our DNA. We can forge our own (skin) success, and that makes me weak at the knees.

Five commandments from the beauty coach

1. Eat your skincare . . .

The skin and hair are the body's window display, and food has an undeniable role in a beauty routine. Beauty food has long-term effects that cosmetic products, with few exceptions, can rarely match. All of the recipes in this book are designed to optimize the skin's well-being. Glossy Rapunzel hair, strong nails, and a healthy body will probably come along with that. Love bomb the body from the inside and the window display will be a polished delight.

2. . . . but complement with hard-core products

The beauty industry churns out a lot of products that are phenomenally good, but the marketing is sometimes padded with fluff. Take various nonpatented "complexes" with pseudoscientific made-up names ("ProYouthFX complex") with a pinch of salt. Some ingredients that really work, however, can be found on page 14. Beauty food + proven effective skincare = magic (although it's actually not magic at all, but instead pure science and chemistry). Regular trips to the skin therapist for a chemical peel or other in-depth treatments are also terrific.

BEAUTY FACT

Take Internet warnings on ingredients with a pinch of salt. Social media sites are overflowing with myths about the hazards of synthetic ingredients. The cosmetics industry is regulated, and you would have to drink products to reach potentially harmful doses. Even a strawberry has substances that could be seen as additives in another food. Natural is good but is not always the most effective in skincare, especially for sensitive skin that can react to essential oils.

3. Create a rainbow

The colors of fruit and vegetables (and salmon) are powerful antioxidants that work hard to protect your beauty from saboteurs, such as ultraviolet (UV) rays, pollutants, and stress. Mix and match the colors of the rainbow and you'll get all the vitamins and antioxidants needed for optimum glow. Also choose wholesome fats so fat-soluble vitamins can be absorbed by the body. Beauty food is not rocket science. Just eat colorfully and you've got it. Think of your favorite eye shadow palette—its beauty lies in the color spectrum.

4. Think addition, not restriction

Beauty food is about including a lot of beauty-affirming products to your diet, not about bans or food anxiety. Give the finger to restrictive diets and instead focus on filling each plate with as much beauty food as you can—the rest will work itself out. And keep in mind that Rome was not built in a day. Nor did Rome collapse if the occasional few rocks were laid crookedly.

5. Feed your soul

The most soul-destroying thing I've ever tried out was the 5:2 diet. I was working at an advertising agency in Copenhagen and this fasting diet spread like wildfire across the office. I felt like I would be cut off from those who ATE FOOD, but I tried it. The result: The calorie app made me anxious and the hunger was horrible. And, really, how COOL was it to have a zero-calorie lunch of nothing but raw bell pepper? It lasted a day. Feed yourself the things that make your soul happy. Wine, good food with fun friends, chocolate, or whatever it may be. We are beauty junkies, not ascetics. (Note: If you like 5:2, I obviously have no objections. But MY soul cried.)

Beauty biology
Skin—how it works

Before we dive into the recipes, here's
a quick course in the biology of the
skin. I promise not to bore you, but
there are some basic things we need
to grasp to understand why we eat
beauty food. The workings inside the
skin are somewhat like a video game,
with different characters to be fed,
guided, or stopped before they
do damage (I'm looking at you,
free radicals—see page 156 for
more on these beauty criminals).

1. Epidermis aka The raincoat

The outermost skin layer is the body's built-in raincoat (think of it as a condom, if you want) that prevents water, ultraviolet (UV) rays, dirt, harmful microorganisms, and other unwanted guests from entering our bodies. The epidermis consists of layers of different cell types, including pigment-producing melanocytes that supervise shades of skin color, dots and spots, immune cells, and keratinocytes.

The keratinocytes are preprogrammed to travel to the stratum corneum (the outermost layer of the epidermis), where they die and shed after about 30 days in a young person. The natural cell renewal process is remarkable, but that is a tragic destiny for a skin cell. However, the process takes longer the older we become, so we can assist those cells that are piling up by cleansing dull, dying cells with skin peels. Certain steps of the cell renewal process result in luster and give what is commonly called a "fresh complexion." Many of us experience dry skin, however, especially in winter or after air travel, which occurs when the stratum corneum is dehydrated. Skin peels and a lot of moisturizer are the only solutions. People with oily skin or acne might attempt to dry out their skin, but this is best avoided, because it triggers the sebaceous glands to produce even more sebum. Dead skin cells clog pores, and trapped oil is a gold mine for acne bacteria. Moisture makes all skin types feel good.

Serums lock in moisture and other ingredients better than creams, and they are a must in every ambitious skincare routine. Invest in a moisturizer that you can drench your face with during the day, and relax with a hydrating mask a few times a week (I love sleep masks that marinate the skin in moisture during the night).

For a happy epidermis:
Beauty food, sunscreen with a minimum SPF of 30, regular peels, products containing vitamin C and antioxidants, and plenty of moisture and barrier-enhancing creams.

2. Dermis
aka The mattress

I know, nobody wants to be called a mattress, but the dermis wears that name with pride. It holds two amazing fiber proteins, collagen and elastin, aiding the skin's padding and springiness. Elastin is the rubber band protein that supplies tension and flexibility, but it weakens over the years to make frown lines more stubborn. Collagen accounts for 80 percent of the skin and makes it look full and as smooth as a peach, but somewhere at about the age of 30, collagen begins to break down, and after 40 years old the decay accelerates. We can't stop time, but we can cheat the beauty saboteurs that attack our collagen and elastin supplies. Beauty food, in combo with good skincare and a sensible lifestyle, reverses the trend by activating collagen formation and postponing the day when the dermis becomes a floppy dormitory mattress. Instead, we are rewarded with a mattress worthy of a luxery hotel suite.

In the dermis, there are also sweat glands, hair follicles, and sebaceous glands, which produce oil that lubricates the skin. Sometimes they become overproductive and then we get pimples. Here, too, live blood vessels, which in some of us are super-reactive. Basically, there is a lot going on in the dermis, 24 hours a day.

For a happy dermis:
Beauty food, sunscreen, deep-penetrating serums with active ingredients, such as retinol, vitamin C, alpha hydroxy acids (AHAs), and peptides.

3. Hypodermis
aka The reservoir

At the bottom of the skin, we find this camera-shy layer that controls our body temperature and acts as a shock absorber. Here, water and fat are stored, but there are also connective tissues that attach the skin to the muscles. If our muscles are tight (from stress, for instance), the skin is affected and loosens (as a jaw grinder, I am painfully aware of this). The phenomenon of "facial fitness" has exploded in recent years. This involves exercising muscles and feeding them with the right things to make the skin as tight as a pair of gym leggings.

For a happy hypodermis:
Beauty food, less stress, massage, and/or LPG treatments.

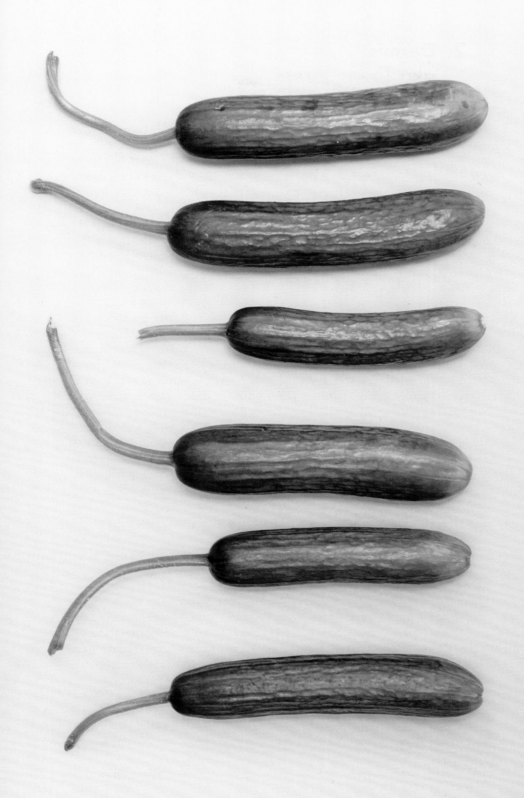

Little beauty parlor

The beauty world is full of difficult words. Don't worry, here we have a skincare nerd's most important terms.

ALPHA HYDROXY ACIDS (AHAS)

Acid sounds like something that would eat away your face (remember Samantha's burned face in *Sex and the City*?), but not in this case. Acids in products for home use are effective but harmless. It's only the dead skin cells that are polished away, and we don't want them anyway. The most common group of acids used for chemical peels is the AHA family. Included in this group are lactic acid, glycolic acid, mandelic acid, and various fruit acids. AHAs wipe away dull dead skin cells so that our chosen skin serum can accomplish its magic without obstacles. They also have proven effects on dryness, lines and superficial wrinkles, acne, moisture levels, old sun damage, and the skin's important cell renewal process.

Which AHA to use depends on the results you seek and the sensitivity of your skin. Lactic acid is great for dry and sensitive skin, while the more deep-penetrating glycolic acid takes care of lines, dryness, and sun damage on a deeper level. Mandelic acid is great for dryness, sun damage, and acne, and is so mild that it's usually fine for sensitive skin.

BETA HYDROXY ACID (BHA)

Also called salicylic acid, this is the best friend of sensitive yet oily and acne-prone skin. It loosens oil from clogged pores and vacuums up sebum and dead skin cells—pore-cleansing masks can't compete. A good choice for reactive skin.

VITAMIN C (ASCORBIC ACID)

A luster hunter's best friend. It is absorbed through the application of serums and creams, and is effective for both the epidermis and dermis. Vitamin C smooths the skin tone, lightens pigmentation, increases collagen production, and gives clarity and glow—like having a spotlight shining under the skin. In addition, its antioxidant properties counteract air pollution. I use vitamin C serum daily to outsmart Stockholm's attempt to sabotage my skin. Be sure to buy vitamin C products in airtight bottles, because oxygen destroys its effects.

HYALURONIC ACID (HA)

Produced in your own body, it can bind a thousand times its own weight in water. Using a serum with hyaluronic acid is like directing a hose at your skin. If a product lists "sodium hyaluronate" in the ingredients, the molecule is small enough to penetrate deep into the skin. On the other hand, "sodium hyaluronate cross polymer" works on the skin's surface, giving a plumping effect. This acid makes your skin go hahaha.

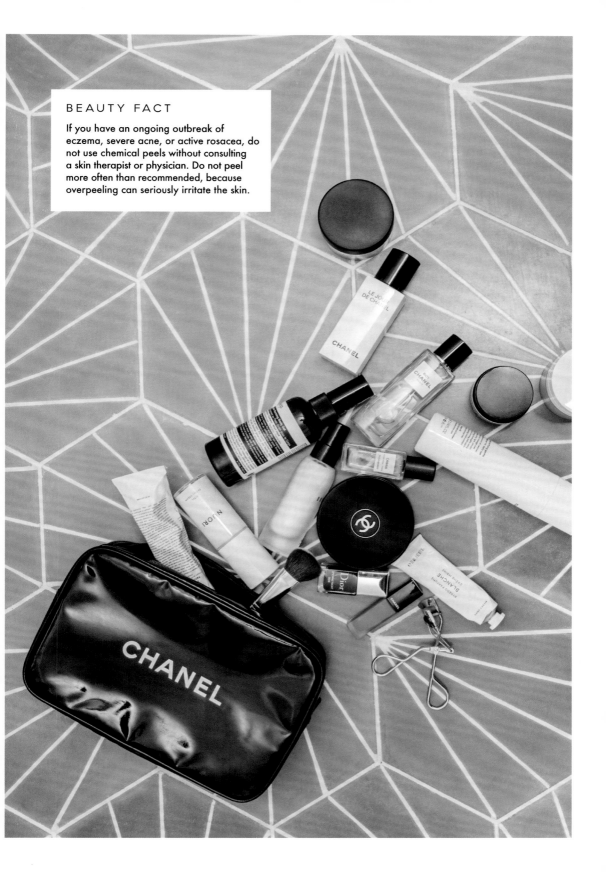

BEAUTY FACT

If you have an ongoing outbreak of eczema, severe acne, or active rosacea, do not use chemical peels without consulting a skin therapist or physician. Do not peel more often than recommended, because overpeeling can seriously irritate the skin.

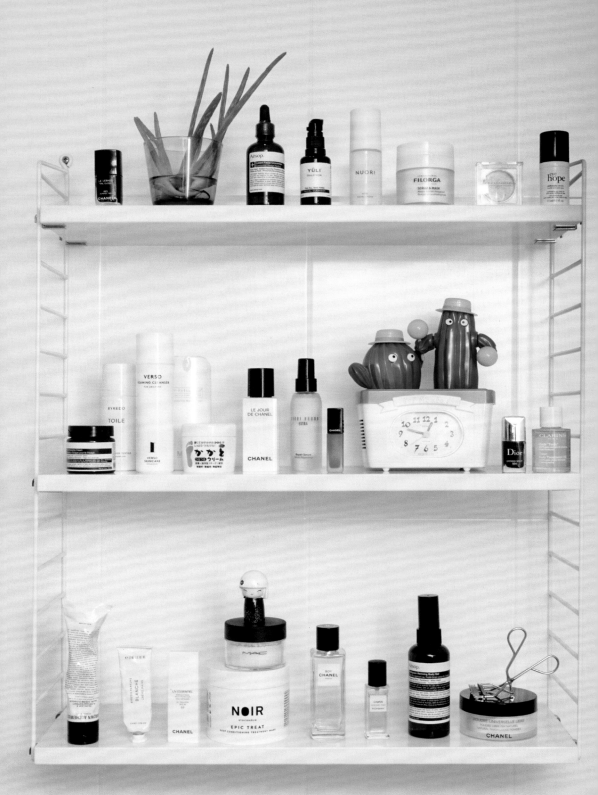

NIACINAMIDE (VITAMIN B₃)

If you are plagued by enlarged pores, you should bring niacinamide into your life. Also an effective vitamin for strengthening sensitive skin and erasing signs of aging. It has an anti-inflammatory effect, which can relieve acne. Like an ibuprofen for the skin!

PEPTIDES

The building blocks of protein, these short chains of amino acids can be used in several clever ways in skincare. Peptides can help the skin to repair itself from external damage and accelerate collagen production so that the skin eventually becomes as firm and as smooth as a freshly ironed shirt.

RETINOL

A form of vitamin A, retinol is one of skin research's most proven and beloved substances. This rock star of the dermatology office is a universal medicine against almost everything. A strong form (tretinoin) is often prescribed to acne patients, while retinol products sold over the counter strengthen thin skin, increase collagen production, reduce lines and wrinkles, and calm occasional outbreaks. Retinol has a cell-communicating effect, which may cause a dull, old skin cell to act like a young kid. How cool is that! New-generation retinol, r-Retinoate, does not cause as much irritation as retinol typically does. It might also be listed in a product's ingredients under names such as retinyl palmitate and retinal. Always wear sunscreen if you are using retinol.

SERUM

The difference between a serum and a cream is that a serum goes deeper into the skin and contains a higher concentration of active ingredients. Serums are a must in your beauty routine if seeking results. Creams take care of the outer barrier and protect it, while a serum is the worker ant that dives into the mine well-stocked with paraphernalia (often filled with one or more of the ingredients in this list).

SUN PROTECTION FACTOR (SPF)

The use of skin products with a sun protection factor (SPF) is by far the best insurance against wrinkles, saggy skin, and pigment stains, but also against the dreaded skin cancer. Skin experts often call SPF products the world's best antiaging tools, because they prevent all of the devastating effects of the sun. Choose so-called wide-spectrum sunscreen that stops both UVA and UVB radiation. A sun filter is either physical, where minerals, such as zinc oxide or titanium dioxide, lie like a mirror on the skin's surface and reflect away the sun's evil rays, or chemical. Chemical sun filters enter the skin, where they absorb dangerous radiation. Some brands mix the two.

SPF foundation rarely provides enough protection for the simple reason that we don't use as much as is needed for full protection. Nowadays, you can find sun protection creams of the so-called city-type, which don't smear or clash with makeup. Choose at least SPF 30 for everyday use, and SPF 50 in the summer or when on vacation.

The beauty saboteurs (and how to outsmart them)

Our poor skin doesn't have it easy. Everyday life is filled with beauty saboteurs that threaten its well-being. However, you can employ an internal security guard to kindly but firmly reject unwanted guests—damage-minimizing beauty foods and effective skincare products will hold down the fort.

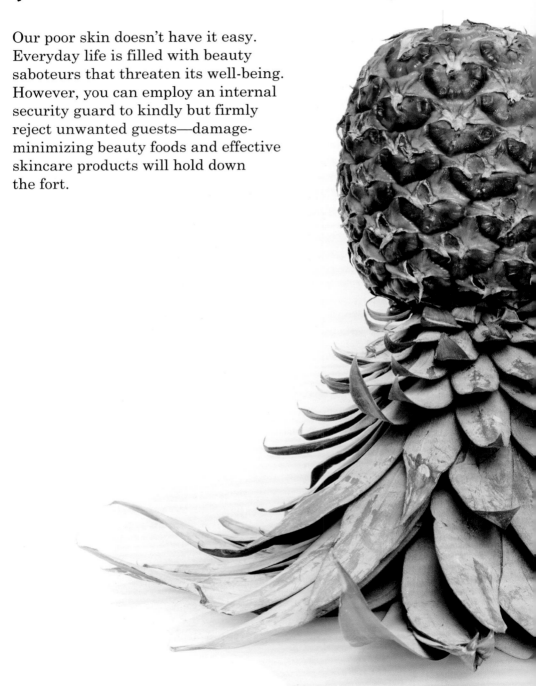

1. Sun

Keep in mind that chilling out in a deckchair can actually cause trauma! For the skin, that's exactly what it does. Getting a tan is a recipe for inflammation and negative skin processes. Every time we get sunburned, damage occurs in the skin's DNA, which eventually appears as wrinkles and discoloration. The risk of skin cancer also increases, no matter how much we'd like to ignore that.

Sun damage is stored in the skin's memory, so sunburn in our youth affects our skin's appearance later in life. The good thing is that the damage can be repaired, but, more important, it can be prevented by simply eating colorful vegetables and fatty fish (preferably in combination with using skincare products that promise to repair DNA damage in the cells).

Sun protection every day is a must to protect your skin against harmful rays, even in wintertime. Clothing gives full protection, but, for the face, a cream with a SPF of 30 is a year-round essential.

2. Sugar

Beauty food is about everything we should eat, not what we should avoid, as dictated by diets that appeal to our fears. However, there is an elephant in the room, namely white sugar. If we constantly feed the body white sugar and fast-release (white) carbohydrates, a bodily reaction called glycation occurs. Sugar molecules then bind to protein molecules to form an end product that is appropriately called an advanced glycation end (AGE) product. The body takes up a defensive position and forms inflammations that cause collagen and elastin to harden, clump up, weaken, and break down. Then wrinkles will appear.

White sugar and carbohydrates have also been shown to trigger outbreaks in acne-prone individuals. However, whole-grain carbs and fruit do not all have the same devastating effects, so there's no need to become militant about a low-carb, high-fat diet. Eating a little sugar every now and then doesn't destroy your complexion, especially if you are otherwise guzzling collagen-stimulating and anti-inflammatory beauty foods. My best advice is to choose slow-release carbohydrates as often as you can.

3. Stress

It's actually not only Murphy's Law that makes the skin go bananas just before a wedding or on the first day of a new job. In the midst of a life crisis, rebellious skin adds insult to injury. Stress triggers inflammatory processes that can lead to flare-ups, increased sensitivity, rashes, and pimples. When life gets stressful, we tend to amplify our anxieties about dieting, eating low-fat, drinking too much wine, smoking, or whatever it may be. Stress can also imbalance hormones and jump-start overactive sebum production, which leads to pimples. For me, when stress becomes overwhelming, I get a lovely cocktail of pimples and rashes around the mouth, itchy eczema on the forearms, and often develop an intolerance of the skincare products that I usually get on fine with.

A number of years ago, I was on the brink of burnout, with nutritional deficiency, hormonal chaos, and acne. One of the first homework assignments I received from my cognitive-behaviorial therapist was to eat real food three times each day, and to feel free to eat cooked food, comfort food. This book contains a lot of anti-inflammatory recipes that feed both body and soul. At home in the bathroom cabinet, sort through all your active products and use only the most basic ones, such as mild cleansers and those that moisturize. Less is more when your life is a mess.

4. Dirt

New research has formed a connection between air pollutants and inflammatory conditions in the skin, such as rosacea, eczema, and acne. The air of big cities is a hotbed of skin-ravaging particles and free radicals. But even small-town folks aren't safe—everyday items, such as photocopiers, generate so-called particulate matter, which interferes with the skin's DNA and accelerates signs of aging, such as discoloration and wrinkles, as well as worsens existing skin conditions. That alone makes you want to isolate yourself from everything.

Before you panic and buy an oxygen tank or cabin in the woods, a cure exists and it is the "antioxidant." Beauty food combined with vitamin C serum and antioxidant-rich creams or oils rescue city/office skin from trauma. I have an antioxidant-enriched moisturizer on my desk and it's great. Skin wins against exhaust fumes, 1–0.

5. Roasting

When it came to my attention that charred food accelerates an array of inner mischief, I felt really fed up. I love crispy burned edges, blackened barbecue food, and roasted things. But sometimes life is a witch. Aggressively heated foods help to create advanced glycation end (AGE) substances in the body, which accelerate signs of aging, such as loose skin, lines, and discoloration, and trigger inflammations that jinx your health. Ouch!

The worst in the class is red meat, but vegetables aren't safe either from chemical reactions. Instead of ditching the barbecue, minimize damage with a large, colorful salad and lovely fresh antioxidant-rich side dishes. During nonbarbecuing season, sauté, steam, or poach as often as possible instead of aggressively heating and charring food. Slow cooking is glow cooking!

Special place of honor: the cigarette

At the beginning of my career as a beauty foodie, I smoked like a chimney, and every Monday, I combated a fragment of the weekend's smoking by eating beauty food in large amounts. Every weekend you could find me in one of Tokyo's many karaoke rooms with a microphone in one hand and a Vogue menthol in the other. And let's not even discuss the trauma that I, as a journalism student at art school in London, exposed my skin to during the first three years of the 2000s. Artists with brooding souls, we smoked in the corridors, at home, at bars and clubs, and everywhere in between.

At the same time, it's normal that young people are not thinking about skin decay at their age. But a few years before I reached the age of 30, I realized I had been mistreating my insides with tar and nicotine for too long, and that it was time to stop if I didn't want to turn into a gray leather bag. I enjoy smoking at a party now and then, because it's just a drop in the ocean (and can be heavenly), but habitual smokers can look forward to the following: increased tendency for acne, premature aging, loose skin, wrinkles and discoloration, prematurely thinning hair, and a gray, lifeless skin tone. Oh, and yellow nails and teeth as well. The good news is that your skin will improve after just a few weeks without cigarettes.

My skin journey— becoming a beauty junkie

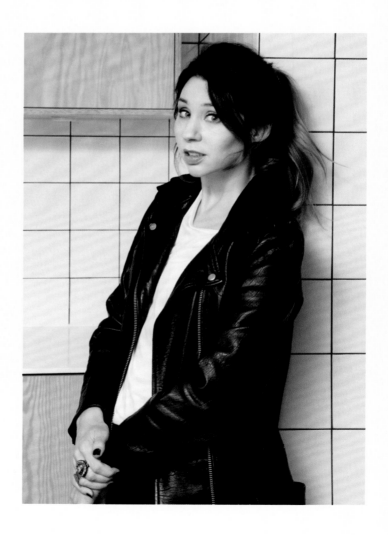

My interest in beauty was born of necessity. I started high school as a living parody of the awkward teenager. Thick, round glasses in a style that my engineer father thought made me look "smart", brutal braces, which gave me the nickname Terminator, an extreme underbite, and hair so crudely colored that you could barely see me on a gray day. Not to forget my constant blushing.

I was painfully far from the early 1990s ideal of a natural beauty with designer jeans, sun-kissed skin, and flowing hair. So after a thousand tears in front of the mirror, I did the only thing I could do— I turned my back on the cool Scandinavian girl concept and went in a completely different direction. Thousands of miles away in the United States, the grunge scene had exploded, and I fell in love with a culture that made room for weird girls like me, even celebrated them. Hair dye and makeup opened the door to the world of taking control of my own look. Instead of being limited by my appearance, I could invent a new version of myself with black eyeliner and cans of hair dye from the local punk store.

Whoever says that makeup is just about superficiality and surfaces has never understood the power of something that gives you the ability and freedom to control your own appearance. A heavy celebration of "natural beauty" and the shaming of makeup users is snobby elitism at its highest level. For those who won the beauty lottery, it's easy to bombard Instagram with no makeup selfies and enlightened quotes, but for us others, the bathroom cabinet holds unmatched possibilities. Which takes us to the next topic close to my heart: the skin.

Skin Chaos No. 1: Eczema

So, I had my game plan and a look that made me feel good. Then the unimaginable happened—I was banned from using makeup. Here's why: I'm atopic and since childhood have had eczema in the bends of my arms and legs. But in the beginning of my second year of high school, something happened. Severe eczema spread around my eyes and mouth. I was confronted with itchy red elephant skin front and center on my face. At times, the eczema spread to my mouth and bled.

I felt uncomfortable, sad, and ugly. My dermatologist brutally zipped shut my makeup bag, so to speak, and I received a depressingly brief list of products that I had the green light to use. To pour salt on the wound, I couldn't use contact lenses for a while either. Glasses, straight bangs, and a red-toned complexion like a character from *Pulp Fiction*, I looked more like a sixteenth-century aristocrat than the cool indie girl I wanted to be. During this period, my dad lived in Hong Kong and worked in medical technology. His Chinese doctor friends came to my rescue and sent me herbs and pills, and I still have no idea what they contained. Sacks of grass-scented green tea were shipped to our little kitchen at my home in Sweden, and something must have worked in my body, because my skin calmed down and I could slowly but surely open the makeup bag again. However, I still had flare-ups of eczema in the bends of my legs and arms, and a wide range of ailments, such as anxiety, swollen stomach, and chronic urinary tract infections, that drew me into an eternal spiral of antibiotics, cures, and a feeling of having gained the world's most worn-out body. You're probably wondering why I'm mentioning all this when it comes to skin? Well, because everything is connected. At the age of 23, I found out that I have a particularly underactive thyroid gland, and it was clearly the main villain in the drama. The skin is a complex window display for our complex bodies.

Skin Chaos No. 2: Acne

At the age of 33, it was time for the next ordeal. Several months after I stopped taking birth control pills, my skin became a sludge of sebum and despair. Red dots emerged all over my cheeks and forehead, some bulging, others like ant bites. Pores as big as craters opened on and around my nose. Sebum erupted and penetrated through concealers and makeup. I was despondent.

A truly stressful existence as a copywriter in a tough advertising agency combined with the mission of a freelance beauty editor at a prestigious fashion magazine added extra fuel to the fire (oh, and then there are the small details of being the mother of a toddler and someone's wife, too—the life of a modern woman). For half a year, I blew through the market's most hyped and exposed products, but because the reason for the chaos was internal, they helped only briefly. I went to a dermatologist and got proper medication and strong creams that nearly made half my face fall off. At the same time, I cleaned up my everyday life. I realized that I'd been living too fast for too long, and my wonderful cognitive-behaviorial therapist helped me to slow down and calm my hyperstressed system. And I started to eat. Proper food that had to be chewed and that took time to eat—not only raw food snacks and juices for "lunch," which, at an advertising agency, meant a 15-minute break that left you with desperate cravings for dessert. With acne medicine, more sensible eating habits, and a total lifestyle makeover, I finally had my skin situation under control and—although it felt pretty tedious—I was able to turn things around.

I was also lucky enough to find a skin therapist who did amazing things with acid treatments and gave me result-orientated products to play around with at home. During this period, I took vitamin B5 supplements, B12, hormone-balancing evening primrose oil, and probiotics. But I felt pretty bad. Skin problems don't stop at the skin. They find their way far into the soul and self-esteem. And acne is so horribly common. Several of my beauty editor colleagues have skin problems. I think you almost have to have skin problems to become a real beauty journalist. It helps you respect the enormous importance of skin in your sense of well-being.

If you're reading this and in the midst of your own intense skin chaos, I would like to remind you of two things. First, skin problems are not shameful; they're human. It's your body trying to tell you something, and—I promise—you can fix it. Second, save valuable time and money by making an appointment to see a skin therapist or dermatologist instead of experimenting with a thousand creams at home. And I hope that the recipes in this book can be one of the pieces of the puzzle on your road to recovery.

But they are only that, a small saving grace. Please remember, I'm a beauty journalist (and professional glow hunter), not a scientist, dietitian, physician, or prophet. And even if I were, there are, in all honesty, no absolute truths in nutrition. New insights emerge constantly and old truths are reconsidered. This book is neither a textbook nor religious writing, but instead (I hope) an inspiring guide that makes you want to look at what's happening in your kitchen with fresh eyes.

Drink your skincare

Juices, smoothies, milk shakes, and other beauty elixirs

Become a beauty mixologist! The blender is central to my skincare routine. Vegetables and fruit are fantastic for the skin, and, when blended, nutrients are immediately absorbed by the body. The blender chews up the food for us, so all we need to do is lean back and wait for an incoming tornado of nutrients that works wonders to maximize the well-being of our skin. I find an almost perverse pleasure in visualizing how all these good things are pushed into my cells and turned into a magic glow while I'm lying on the couch and lazily watching Netflix. It's really incredible to devour a whole salad in one drink—with the only drawback of kale stuck between your teeth.

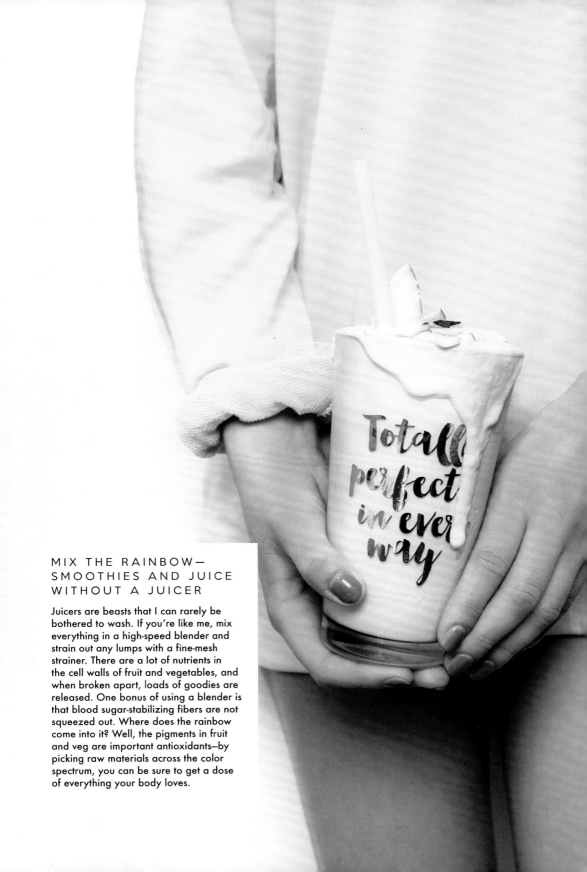

MIX THE RAINBOW— SMOOTHIES AND JUICE WITHOUT A JUICER

Juicers are beasts that I can rarely be bothered to wash. If you're like me, mix everything in a high-speed blender and strain out any lumps with a fine-mesh strainer. There are a lot of nutrients in the cell walls of fruit and vegetables, and when broken apart, loads of goodies are released. One bonus of using a blender is that blood sugar-stabilizing fibers are not squeezed out. Where does the rainbow come into it? Well, the pigments in fruit and veg are important antioxidants—by picking raw materials across the color spectrum, you can be sure to get a dose of everything your body loves.

Green

Cucumber, avocado, lime, leafy greens, mango, and mint.

1 GLASS
1 cucumber
½ avocado or ½ cup frozen, diced avocado
juice of 1–2 limes
a generous handful of mint
about 1 cup baby spinach or kale
½ banana, sliced and frozen
⅔ cup frozen mango chunks
splash of plant-based milk, if required

Peel the cucumber if it's not organic. Cut the cucumber and avocado into pieces, then blend with the other ingredients in a high-speed blender until smooth. Add a splash of milk if the consistency is too thick.

BEAUTY BONUS NO. 1

Dark green leafy vegetables are a cocktail of vitamins and minerals that are indispensable for beautiful skin. The antioxidant beta-carotene protects the skin against external stresses.

Purple

Blackberries, vanilla, and red beets.

1 GLASS
1¼ cups frozen blackberries
½ teaspoon vanilla powder
¼ cup red beet juice or ½ cooked red beet, cubed
1¼ cups plant-based milk

Blend all the ingredients in a high-speed blender until smooth.

BEAUTY BONUS NO. 2

Red and purple fruits and vegetables get their vibrant color from anthocyanins, which are an entire army of age- and inflammation-fighting molecules. Vitamin C accelerates collagen formation.

Blue

Blueberries, almond butter, banana, vanilla, cinnamon, and cardamom.

1 GLASS
1¼ cups frozen blueberries
2 tablespoons almond butter
1 teaspoon vanilla powder
1 teaspoon ground cardamom
1 teaspoon ground cinnamon
1 banana, sliced and frozen
1¼ cups plant-based milk

Blend all the ingredients in a high-speed blender until smooth.

BEAUTY BONUS NO. 3

Fat-soluble vitamins need—surprise—fat to be absorbed by the body, so using nut butter, avocado, or coconut oil in a smoothie maximizes the beauty effects.

Pink

Strawberries, peanut butter, vanilla, and goji berries.

1 GLASS
1 tablespoon goji berries
1⅓ cups fresh or frozen (partly defrosted) strawberries
1 tablespoon peanut butter
½ teaspoon vanilla powder
1¼ cups plant-based milk

Soak the goji berries in water for about 20 minutes. Drain, then blend the berries with the other ingredients in a high-speed blender until smooth.

BEAUTY BONUS NO. 4

Strawberries are full of vitamin C, which protects against external beauty saboteurs and gives a boost to collagen.

Red

Red beets, lingonberries, and raspberries.

1 GLASS
**1 cup red beet juice (juice yourself
  or buy prepared organic juice)**
⅓ cup frozen lingonberries
½ cup frozen raspberries
½ cup coconut water

Blend the beet juice with the other ingredients in a high-speed blender until smooth.

Yellow

Lemon, orange, mango, and ginger.

1 GLASS
1-inch piece of fresh ginger
juice of 1–2 lemons
juice of 1 orange
1½ cups frozen mango chunks
1 cup plant-based milk

Peel the ginger, then slice into smaller pieces. Blend with the other ingredients in a high-speed blender until smooth.

Orange

Orange, carrot, mango, sea buckthorn, turmeric, and ginger.

1 GLASS
2 carrots
1-inch piece of fresh ginger
juice of 2 oranges
1 cup frozen mango chunks
⅔ cup frozen sea buckthorn berries
pinch of ground turmeric
**½ cup coconut water or water, plus extra
  if required**

Peel the carrots and ginger, then slice into smaller pieces. Blend with the other ingredients in a high-speed blender until smooth, adding more coconut water or water as needed.

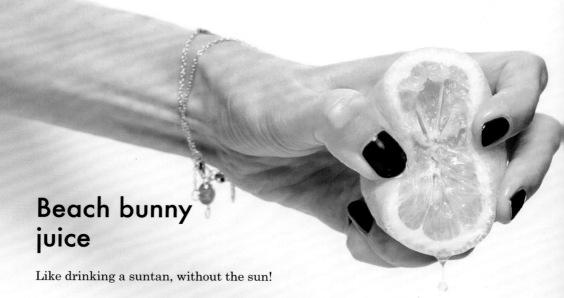

Beach bunny juice

Like drinking a suntan, without the sun!

1 GLASS
5 carrots
2 lemons
1-inch piece of fresh ginger
1⅔ cups frozen mango chunks

Peel the carrots, lemons, and ginger, then push them through a raw juice extractor. Transfer the juice to a bowl and add the mango, then blend with a handheld blender (or use a high-speed blender) until velvety smooth.

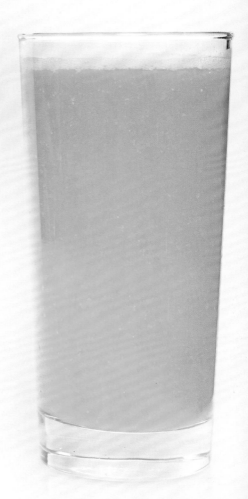

BEAUTY
BONUS NO. 8

Carrot and mango are bursting with beta-carotene, which enhances your sun-kissed tone and gives the skin's natural sunscreen extra muscles. Start boosting the beta-carotene in your daily menu ten weeks before a vacation in the sun.

Summer, sun, and liquid sunscreen—prepare for a vacation from within

As a child of the 1980s sunscreen-skeptical Hawaiian Tropic culture, I see it as one of my life's purposes to recover what I can of my skin. And it is actually possible to mitigate the sun's harmful effects and repair parts of already damaged goods.

Prepare for a vacation in the sun by eating beauty food, which provides extra protection against beauty-sabotaging rays, and applying creamy sunscreen, then you will be rewarded both on a long-term basis and more immediately with a more beautiful tan that won't peel as soon as you board the flight home. Antioxidants beta-carotene and lycopene boost the skin cells' own defense against sun damage, so before and during the sunny season, fuel up with red, yellow, and orange veggies such as carrot, mango, tomato, and watermelon. The lycopene in tomato is best eaten in heated form, but foods such as watermelon are a better raw source.

IMPORTANT THINGS TO KNOW ABOUT SPF IN SUNSCREEN

Even if we drink 3 quarts of carrot juice a day, we cannot under any circumstances neglect using sunscreen. There isn't a big difference between SPF 50 and 30, but, as a defender of the skin, I say definitely no lower than the latter. I prefer a physical sunscreen, which lets minerals (usually zinc oxide or titanium dioxide) rest on the skin's surface and reflect the sun's evil rays away, like a mirror. This is the best choice for those of us with sensitive, pimple-prone skin (aka "the skin type that God forgot").

Matcha mojito smoothie

A combination of mint, lime, and exotic fruit is your ticket to a sunnier mood. Mix with chlorophyll-packed matcha powder and leafy greens to make a world-class beauty bomb.

1 GLASS
1 cup spinach leaves and/or kale
½ bunch of mint, plus an extra sprig
to decorate
1¼ cups plant-based milk
juice of 2 limes
1 tablespoon yacon syrup (see page 154)
1 teaspoon vanilla powder
1 tablespoon organic matcha powder
1⅔ cups frozen mango or 1 cup frozen
pineapple chunks

Blend the spinach and/or kale, mint, and milk in a high-speed blender until smooth. Add the lime juice, yacon syrup, vanilla, and matcha, then add the mango or pineapple, a little at a time (I usually drop the pieces through the hole in the lid while the blender is still running), and continue to blend until smooth. Pour into a glass and decorate with a sprig of mint.

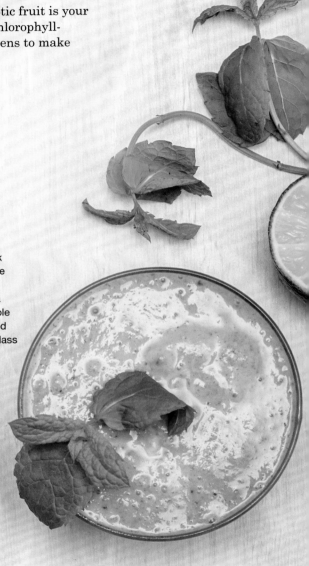

BEAUTY
BONUS NO. 9

Organic matcha powder can be found in health-food stores, well-stocked tea suppliers, and at some pharmacies with a health food section.

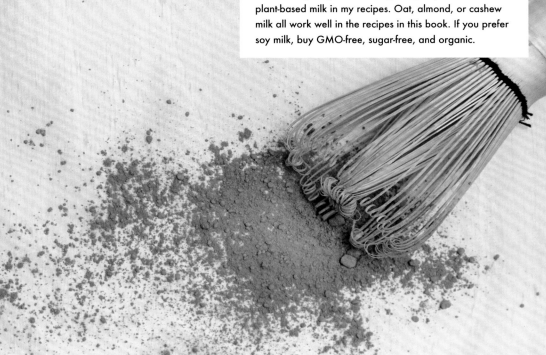

MILK AND BREAKOUTS— WHAT'S THE TRUTH?

Raise your hand if you have woken to a pimply skin crisis after an intense romance with a box of chocolates or a scoop of ice cream. There seems to be some scientific truth that after a chocolate marathon, a pimple fest follows. It's not the cocoa butter but the milk (in good company with the mega beauty saboteur, sugar) that seems to be the culprit. Research shows that there's a link between cow milk and acne. Hormones in the milk, especially highly processed low-fat milk, cause the insulin and growth hormone IGF-1 to skyrocket, and the body responds with increased sebum production, inflammation, and clogged pores, which can lead to pimples. The problem with this study is that it focused on teens with preexisting acne. Plenty of people can guzzle lattes and not have so much as a single blemish. In my case, for several years (packed with partying), I pumped myself full of at least one giant skinny latte and a pint of nonfat frozen yogurt a day without even a trace of a pimple, while later in life, as a raw food vegan, I was struck by an acne crisis associated with birth control pills.

To sum up, how the body handles milk varies on an individual basis, but to be on the safe side and not to encourage any sebaceous glands, I try to stick to plant-based milk in my recipes. Oat, almond, or cashew milk all work well in the recipes in this book. If you prefer soy milk, buy GMO-free, sugar-free, and organic.

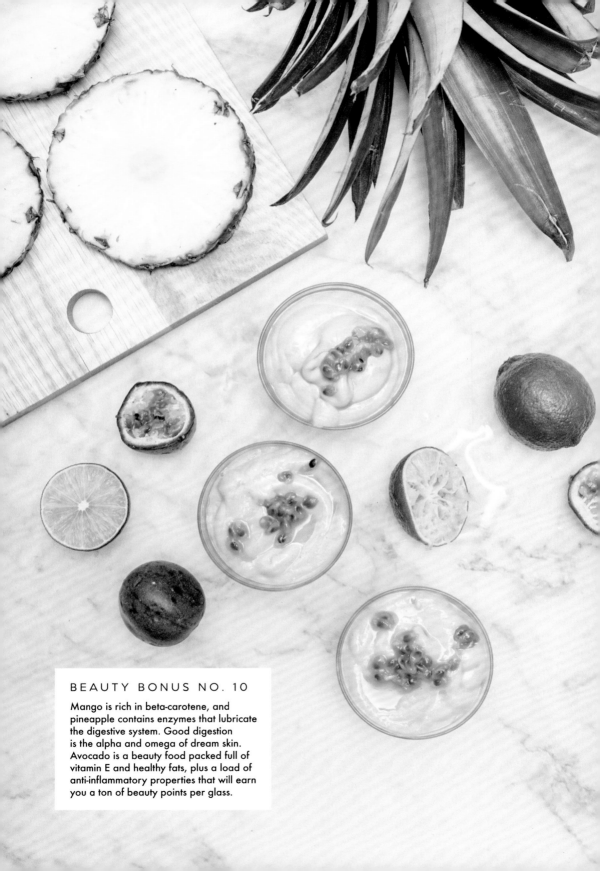

BEAUTY BONUS NO. 10

Mango is rich in beta-carotene, and pineapple contains enzymes that lubricate the digestive system. Good digestion is the alpha and omega of dream skin. Avocado is a beauty food packed full of vitamin E and healthy fats, plus a load of anti-inflammatory properties that will earn you a ton of beauty points per glass.

Poolside pineapple smoothie

Treat your friends to this liquid sunshine or keep it waiting in the refrigerator for yourself. The superbeauty fruit avocado makes a silky smoothie. With this in stock, I go back and forth between the balcony and the refrigerator until I've started to wear out the floor.

1 PITCHER
1 ripe pineapple or 1 cup frozen
   pineapple chunks
2 ripe avocados
2-inch piece of fresh ginger
juice of 3–4 limes
3½–4¼ cups plant-based milk
2⅓ cups frozen mango chunks
1 banana, sliced and frozen

TO DECORATE
passion fruit pulp
toasted coconut chips (optional)

If using fresh pineapple, slice off the top and bottom, then carefully cut away the skin and cut the flesh into pieces. Chop the avocados into pieces. Peel the ginger. Blend the pineapple and avocados with the lime juice, ginger, and milk in a high-speed blender until smooth. Add the frozen mango and banana through the hole in the lid while the machine is running to really whip up the ultimate creaminess. If the mixture becomes too thick to blend, add more milk.

Top off each glass with a little passion fruit pulp and coconut chips before serving.

Milk shakes and coffee drinks

Coffee, chocolate, and banana—three common ingredients for worry wrinkles

Can coffee be a beauty food?

Yes, of course! Both coffee and cacao are loaded with antioxidants. I am such a grumpy morning person that my worries would dig deep in no time without coffee, so I consider coffee as a supporting part of my skincare routine. I'm crazy about coffee in every way. Coffee is therapy! Foamy cappuccino, alert espresso, frosty coffee milk shake, coffee ice cream, mocha mousse, coffee in raw food brownies or chocolate balls , . . you get the idea.

My love for coffee is the reason I have never been on a detox. My firm conviction is that if you live a fairly balanced life and eat beauty food, no strict detox is needed. The body has a built-in cleaning system that handles detoxification wonderfully without needing to buy expensive detox treatments.

What about chocolate?

No beauty routine is complete without cacao. Preferably, it should be raw, and not heated. Eating it raw preserves a whole array of nutrients in the cacao, making it a model ingredient in the beauty pantry. Its sky-high antioxidant content, especially the flavonoids, works hard against the free radicals that age our skin.

Raw cacao also contains tryptophan, which is converted into the happiness hormone serotonin in the body. It's, therefore, no coincidence that we crave chocolate when we feel low, bored, and/or have PMS.

Banana?

This poor yellow fruit has been blacklisted by carbohydrate antagonists and the diet industry, but it's an amazing beauty fruit. Frozen chunks of banana are transformed in a blender into beauty-proofed soft ice cream or a fluffy milk shake, depending on how much milk you add. Here, too, we find the pleasurable amino acid tryptophan. And as I say, that's important for your soul. The skin is the body's window display, and a happy soul leads to happy skin.

Frozen fabuccino

Creamy iced frappuccinos sold at coffee shops are my favorite summertime guilty pleasure, but they're often packed with the beauty saboteur sugar. So I took things into my own hands and made my own beauty-proofed version— a frozen fabuccino!

1 GLASS
1 banana, sliced and frozen
⅔ cup cold coffee or 2 shots of espresso
1 teaspoon vanilla powder
1¼ cup plant-based milk
ice cubes

Blend all the ingredients in a high-speed blender. Drink immediately.

TIP!
Want a sugar-free fabuccino? Replace the banana with a lot of ice and sweeten with a little stevia, if you like. I like stevia drops, which can be found in health-food stores, various pharmacies, and well-stocked grocery stores.

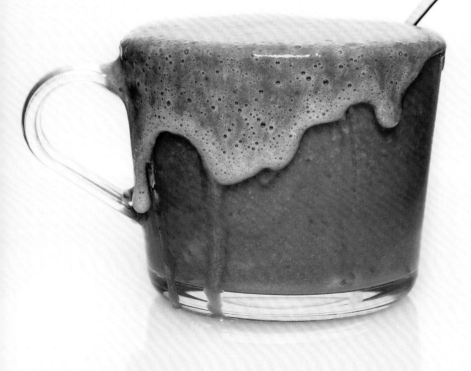

Frozen mochaccino

Coffee and chocolate are concentrated happiness. In this recipe, adjust the sweetness, as well as the chocolate and coffee strength, to your liking. I like it fairly sweet. Mesquite flour (see page 152) is a bit hard to find (one solution is to order online), but it lends a delicious caramel twist.

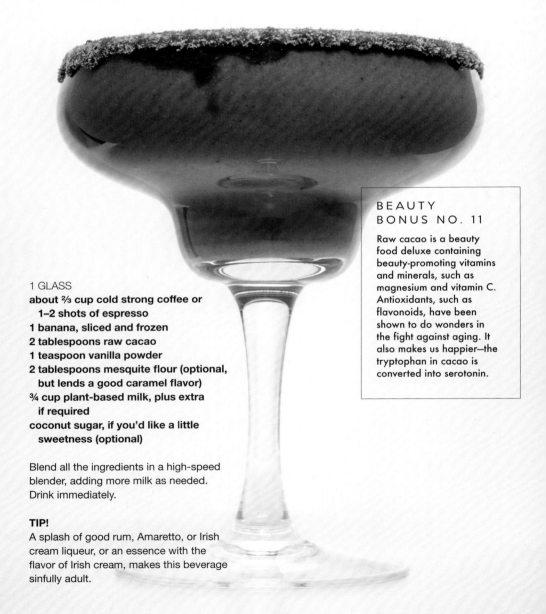

1 GLASS
about ⅔ cup cold strong coffee or
   1–2 shots of espresso
1 banana, sliced and frozen
2 tablespoons raw cacao
1 teaspoon vanilla powder
2 tablespoons mesquite flour (optional,
   but lends a good caramel flavor)
¾ cup plant-based milk, plus extra
   if required
coconut sugar, if you'd like a little
   sweetness (optional)

Blend all the ingredients in a high-speed blender, adding more milk as needed. Drink immediately.

TIP!
A splash of good rum, Amaretto, or Irish cream liqueur, or an essence with the flavor of Irish cream, makes this beverage sinfully adult.

**BEAUTY
BONUS NO. 11**

Raw cacao is a beauty food deluxe containing beauty-promoting vitamins and minerals, such as magnesium and vitamin C. Antioxidants, such as flavonoids, have been shown to do wonders in the fight against aging. It also makes us happier—the tryptophan in cacao is converted into serotonin.

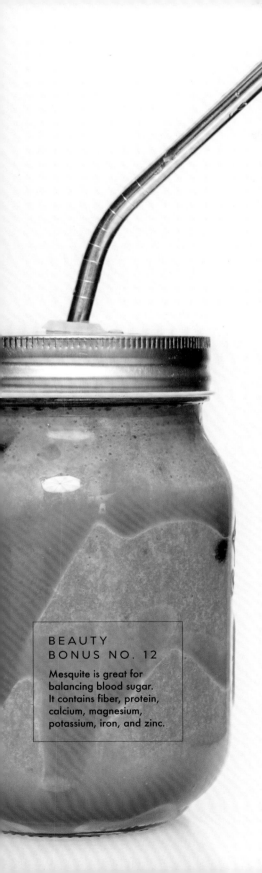

Superfood-spiked caramel shake

For a short time, I had an intensive love affair with bikram yoga. But as a person with a mild phobia of bacteria and other people's bodily fluids, it was a test to stand in downward-facing dog pose next to strange men dripping with sweat. The first time I managed a whole class, I celebrated with an unforgettable icy milk shake. The sweetness of the victory and the shake was almost too much wonderfulness to handle all at the same time. Here's the recipe for it.

1 GLASS
1 large or 2 small bananas, sliced and frozen
2 tablespoons mesquite flour
2 tablespoons yacon syrup
1 teaspoon vanilla powder
1 teaspoon ground cardamom
1⅔ cups plant-based milk

RAW CARAMEL SAUCE (OPTIONAL)
10 dates (preferably medjool)
2 tablespoons plant-based milk,
    plus extra if required
1 teaspoon vanilla powder

If making the sauce, start by pitting the dates, then soak them in water for at least 10 minutes, until soft. Drain, then slice into small pieces. Blend the dates with the milk and vanilla in a small food processor (a blender doesn't work as well) to make a smooth sauce, adding more milk, if necessary. Drizzle the sauce around the edges of a drinking jar or a glass.

Blend the banana, mesquite flour, yacon syrup, vanilla, cardamom, and milk in a high-speed blender until smooth. Pour into the jar or glass.

BEAUTY
BONUS NO. 12

Mesquite is great for balancing blood sugar. It contains fiber, protein, calcium, magnesium, potassium, iron, and zinc.

Peanut-y chocolate caramel milk shake

A healthy homage to Snickers, one of the greatest chocolate bars on earth. Did you know that it's a good idea to indulge in this milk shake at least once each time you have PMS? Well, now you do!

1 GLASS
1 banana, sliced and frozen
1 tablespoon raw cacao
1 tablespoon peanut butter
1 teaspoon vanilla powder
1⅔ cups plant-based milk

TOPPING
Raw Caramel Sauce (see page 39)
peanuts (preferably unsalted)
raw cacao nibs

Blend all the ingredients in a high-speed blender until smooth. Pour into a glass and top off with Raw Caramel Sauce, peanuts, and cacao nibs. For a stronger caramel taste, you can put some of the Raw Caramel Sauce at the bottom of the glass before adding the milk shake.

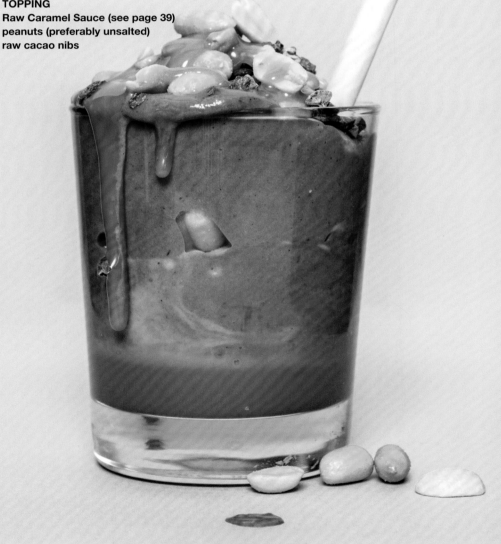

Raw chocolate pudding shake

Like drinking fluffy chocolate pudding. You can read more about yacon syrup on page 154 in the Beautypedia. If you can't find this magical sweetener, liquid coconut nectar works instead and can be found in some well-stocked grocery stores or health-food stores.

1 GLASS
1 avocado
2–3 tablespoons raw cacao
1–2 tablespoons yacon syrup or
 liquid coconut nectar
1 teaspoon vanilla powder
1¼ cups plant-based milk
ice cubes

TO DECORATE
raw cacao nibs

Blend all the ingredients in a high-speed blender until smooth. Top off with cacao nibs.

TIP!
For a more frozen consistency, use frozen diced avocado. You can find it in the frozen foods section of large grocery stores, and it's the most wonderful thing ever.

BEAUTY
BONUS NO. 13

Avocado is the queen of vitamin E and the healthy fatty acids that skin loves.

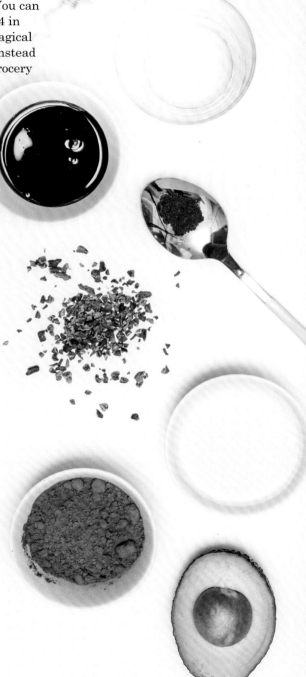

Glow in a bowl

Smoothie bowls, fluff, raw soups, and other cold things in a bowl

Bowl food is soul food. As much as I like partying and celebrating with friends, I love to crawl up on the couch in pajamas and woolly socks with a bowl filled with goodness. If I've had a hearty lunch, in the evenings I often crave just a bowl filled with something cold and creamy. It may be a minty smoothie bowl, an ice-creamy acai bowl, mango fluff, or a raw soup that I can make in about 30 seconds in the blender.

The toppings are half the pleasure. Also, you earn a lot of beauty points, and the beneficial fats help the body to absorb important vitamins. In my kitchen, there are countless glass jars of pumpkin seeds, sunflower seeds, nuts, hemp seeds, goji berries, raw cacao nibs, coconut chips, chia seeds, and so on. The good thing about cooking is that you can make it up as you go: add and take away and customize your bowl from time to time. As I write this, I have on my knee a bowl of banana ice cream flavored with matcha powder and cardamom. And, of course, woolly socks on my feet.

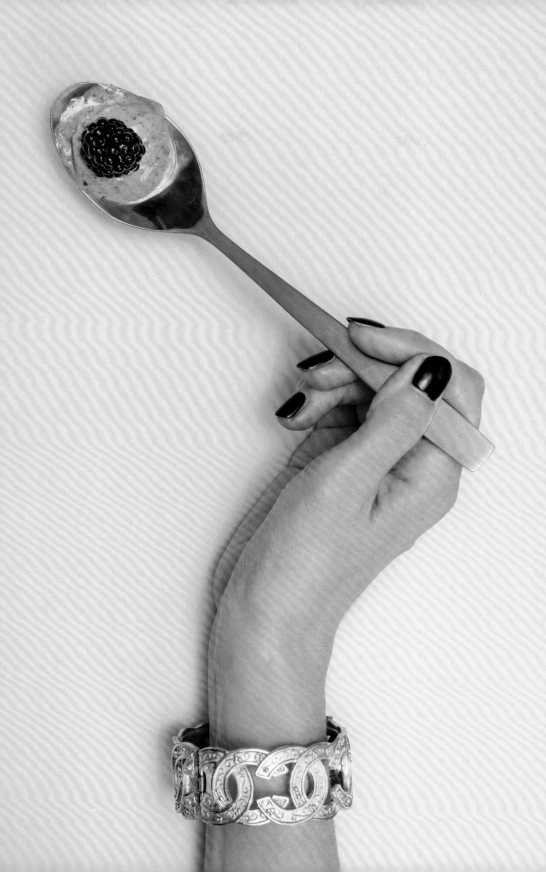

Green beauty bowl

In another life, where each day wasn't a marathon of school drop-offs and managing to arrive at work in a fairly respectable state (I'm happy if I have time to put on mascara), I would make this bowl every morning. Then I would go to yoga and chant "om" until the next meal. But as long as I live a life of Swedish kitchen countertop realism, I'll enjoy it for dinner or a weekend meal. Sweet, sour, eye-catching, and so, so wonderful.

1 PORTION

1 cup baby spinach or kale
juice of 1–2 limes or lemons
½ cup plant-based milk, plus extra if required
1½ cups frozen mango chunks
pinch of vanilla powder
pinch of ground cinnamon
pinch of ground cardamom

Blend all the ingredients until creamy, adding more milk as needed. Top off with whatever you like—I usually pile on soft fruits, seeds, and edible flowers, or goji berries and cacao nibs.

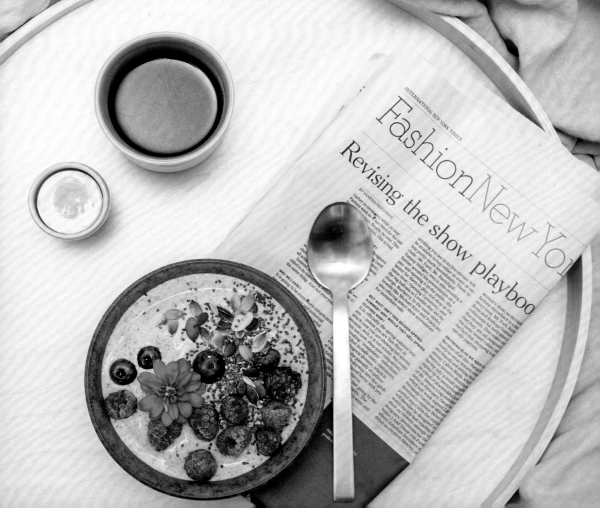

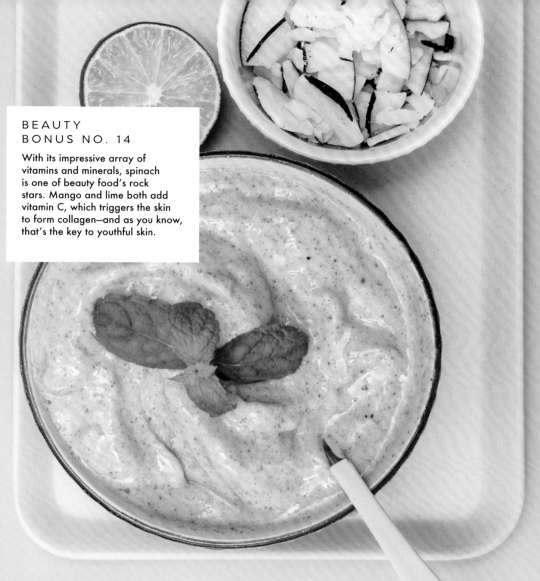

Mojito bowl

Are you allowed to have a frozen mojito
for breakfast? Mint and lime are one
of life's best combinations. You can
find frozen pineapple in well-stocked
grocery stores, but it's fine to use frozen
mango instead. Coconut milk makes
the vacation sensation complete.

1 SERVING
juice of 2 limes
1–2 large handfuls of mint, plus an
   extra sprig to decorate
1 cup baby spinach
½ cup coconut milk or other plant-based milk
1 cup frozen pineapple chunks

TOPPING
fresh coconut pieces

Blend the lime juice, mint, baby spinach, and milk.
Add the pineapple and blend until it reaches the
consistency of sorbet. Decorate with a sprig of
mint and serve with fresh coconut pieces.

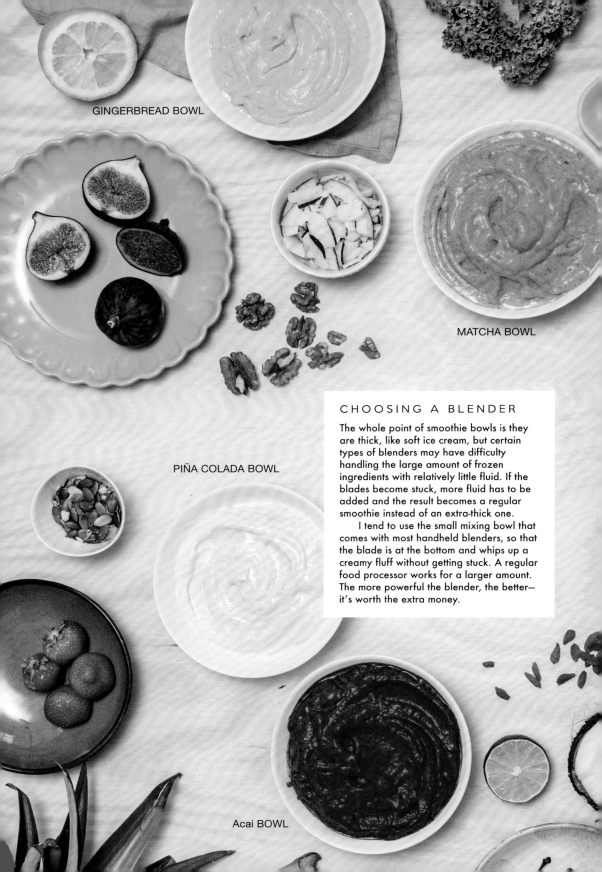

GINGERBREAD BOWL

MATCHA BOWL

PIÑA COLADA BOWL

Acai BOWL

CHOOSING A BLENDER

The whole point of smoothie bowls is they are thick, like soft ice cream, but certain types of blenders may have difficulty handling the large amount of frozen ingredients with relatively little fluid. If the blades become stuck, more fluid has to be added and the result becomes a regular smoothie instead of an extra-thick one.

I tend to use the small mixing bowl that comes with most handheld blenders, so that the blade is at the bottom and whips up a creamy fluff without getting stuck. A regular food processor works for a larger amount. The more powerful the blender, the better—it's worth the extra money.

Gingerbread bowl

I don't know if gingerbread makes you nicer, but without a doubt this smoothie bowl, maxed with anti-inflammatory protein, beta-carotene, and vitamin C, will work extremely hard for your skin. Juice your own carrots or buy freshly pressed juice.

1 SERVING
juice of 1 orange
⅔ cup carrot juice
1 tablespoon peanut butter
½ teaspoon gingerbread spice, plus extra to taste
pinch of vanilla powder
1½ cups frozen mango chunks

Blend all the ingredients until creamy, adding more gingerbread spice, if liked. Serve immediately.

TIP!
If you want to make it even more luxurious, replace the mango with frozen sea buckthorn berries, which contain essential fatty acids that moisturize dry mucous membranes.

Piña colada bowl

Sweet and sour and delicious enough to work as dessert. If having for dessert, use smaller glasses, top off with fresh berries and coconut, and serve immediately. If the coconut milk is overpowering, replace half of it with coconut water.

1 SERVING
1½ cups frozen pineapple chunks
1 cup coconut milk
juice of 2 limes
pinch of vanilla powder

Blend all the ingredients until smooth and fluffy. Serve immediately.

Matcha bowl

Like a green ice cream with extra superpowers! The banana's sweetness balances the bitterness of the matcha, and the spinach adds tons of green beauty points.

1 SERVING
2 bananas, sliced and frozen
1 cup baby spinach
½ cup plant-based milk
½ tablespoon organic matcha powder
pinch of vanilla powder

Blend all the ingredients until the consistency of ice cream. If the blender blades seem stuck, leave the banana slices to defrost for a few minutes before you resume blending. Serve immediately.

Acai bowl

Acai berries can be found in both powdered and frozen puree form. You will want the latter to achieve that ice creamlike consistency.

1 SERVING
3½-oz bag frozen acai puree
1 banana, sliced and frozen
1 cup frozen blueberries
½ cup plant-based milk, plus extra if required
pinch of vanilla powder

Remove the bag of acai puree from the freezer a few minutes before blending, otherwise it will lie there like a block of ice in the blender mixing bowl. Blend all the ingredients until the consistency of sorbet, adding a little extra milk if the blades become stuck. Serve immediately.

TIP!
Top off with traditional acai bowl friends, such as sliced fresh strawberries, sliced banana, coconut shavings, and a dollop of peanut butter.

Fluff—protein-pimped bowls to fuel your glow

The first time I added whey protein powder to a smoothie bowl it was as if the heavens opened. My husband was in an athletic phase (crisis related, linked to being 40 years old) and there were a lot of products around the house designed to boost his newfound identity as a triathlete/ironman/lycra-clad cyclist. I took a scoop from a bag labeled "whey protein," and whoa! Smoothies became a cloud of ice creamlike fluff that almost lifted the blender lid! In addition to the combination of frozen fruit, whey protein is the source of a lot of amino acids that are indispensable building blocks for skin, hair, and muscles.

But—and this is important—be sure not to buy any synthetic whey diluted with sweeteners (strange confectionery flavors give it away), and check the packaging to confirm that the whey comes from grass-fed cows that haven't been pumped full of hormones. It's an absolute must for beauty foodies to be a little snobby about using pure whey protein powder of the finest quality.

Here, I have to inject another strong word of caution. For some people, whey protein may aggravate acne, because it triggers the body's natural growth hormone IGF-1, which can increase oil production. If you notice your fluff bowls causing pimples, replace the whey protein with a protein powder made from pea, hemp, or brown rice, or skip the extra protein entirely. Unfortunately, the fluffiness is lost, but you'll still have a creamy smoothie mixture. Add some sliced, frozen banana and you'll get ice cream.

> **BEAUTY BONUS NO. 15**
>
> Whey protein contains a three-stage rocket of the amino acids cysteine, glycine, and glutamine, which helps the body form superantioxidant glutathione. Cysteine is important for the hair and skin. It also protects against the breakdown of muscle, and we definitely need to remember that our entire face is composed of muscles.

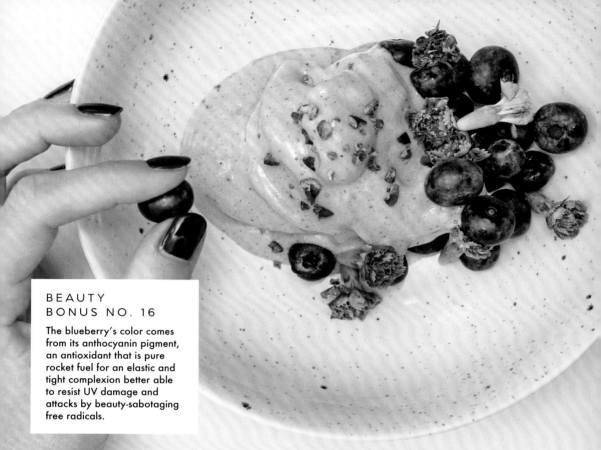

Blueberry, vanilla, and cardamom fluff

If you want to avoid whey protein but still get an ice cream consistency, add a handful of frozen banana pieces instead. Lucuma powder or mesquite flour lend a caramel-like sweetness, but you can omit them if you can't find them. Decorate as you please. I use fresh blueberries, edible flowers, and a sprinkling of cacao nibs for added crunch.

1 SERVING

⅔ cup plant-based milk
1½ cups frozen blueberries
1 tablespoon yacon syrup or coconut nectar,
   plus extra to taste
2 tablespoons vanilla-flavor whey protein powder
pinch of vanilla powder
pinch of ground cardamom
½ tablespoon lucuma powder or mesquite flour
   (see page 152)

Blend all the ingredients until completely smooth, adding more yacon syrup or coconut nectar, if liked. Serve immediately.

Strawberry and lime fluff

A vessel laden with wrinkle-stopping vitamin C and plenty of antioxidants! Frozen strawberries can be a little tough on a blender, so let them defrost a little before getting started.

1 SERVING

⅔ cup plant-based milk
1½ cups frozen (slightly defrosted) strawberries, plus 1 fresh to decorate
juice of 1 lime
2 tablespoons vanilla-flavor whey protein powder
pinch of vanilla powder

Blend all the ingredients in batches until smooth. Decorate with the fresh strawberry and serve.

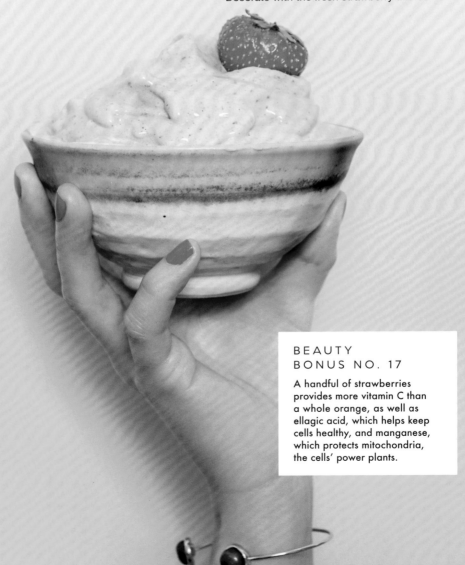

BEAUTY
BONUS NO. 17

A handful of strawberries provides more vitamin C than a whole orange, as well as ellagic acid, which helps keep cells healthy, and manganese, which protects mitochondria, the cells' power plants.

Mango and lemon fluff

Congratulations to readers and their skin, who will enjoy the effects of this tantalizing sweet-and-sour glow bowl. I don't know which will be turning more somersaults—the skin, the mouth, or the soul. Top with fresh or dried fruit, nuts, seeds, even edible flowers, and you'll shed a tear of joy.

1 SERVING
½ cup plant-based milk
1½ cups frozen mango chunks
juice of 1 lemon
2 tablespoons vanilla-flavor whey
   protein powder
pinch of vanilla powder

Blend all the ingredients until smooth and fluffy. Serve immediately.

BEAUTY BONUS NO. 18

Lemon is a bomb of vitamin C. Antioxidants mop up those pesky free radicals, strengthen the immune system, and provide the conditions for a glowing complexion able to cope with external threats.

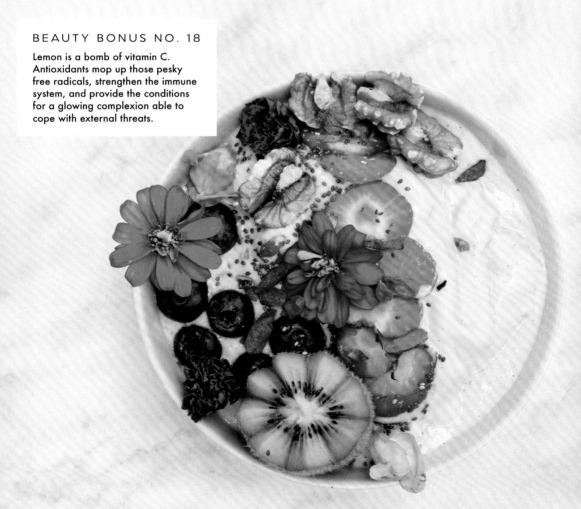

Boost your glow with toppings

Toppings are half the fun of bowl food. Here are my favorites to keep your skin baby soft, springy like a trampoline, and less inviting for invaders, such as free radicals and acne bacteria.

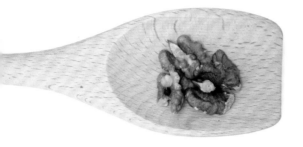

Walnuts

One of the few friends from the plant kingdom containing skin-strengthening omega-3 in the form of alpha-linolenic acid (ALA). A small fistful of walnuts a day helps the skin keep up moisture levels during the winter. Walnuts are also rich in antioxidants.

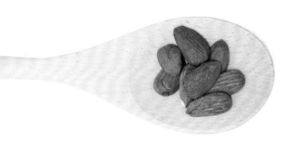

Almonds

Wrinkles beware! The almond boasts one of nature's highest contents of vitamin E, which protects our valuable cell membranes. Think of vitamin E as the police officer that stops free radicals from running amok. Almonds are also rich in magnesium.

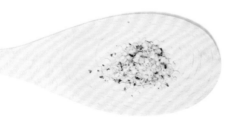

Hemp seeds

These contain all the essential amino acids and an optimal balance between omega-3 and omega-6 fatty acids. The seeds have been shown in studies to relieve dry and eczema-prone skin. Contains the fatty acid GLA, which can balance hormones. Thank you, says the PMS monster.

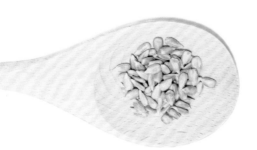

Sunflower seeds

Loaded with vitamin E. In a study where dogs were fed with sunflower seeds and flaxseeds, their coats were shinier after about 14 days.

Raw cacao nibs

Raw cacao is stuffed with superantioxidant flavonoids that protect against external beauty saboteurs and can even produce smoother skin. In a Korean study, cacao flavonoids have been shown to affect the wrinkles and skin firmness of people with moderate signs of aging.

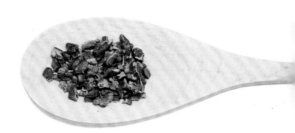

Chia seeds

Each little chia seed has a 20 percent content of the favorite omega-3 fatty acid, which can reduce inflammation and protect against various issues that come with aging. It's a complete protein, with all the building blocks necessary for skin, hair, and nails. It also contains a lot of dietary fiber.

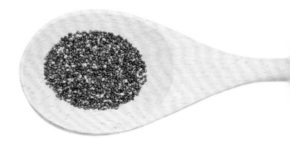

Pumpkin seeds

My favorite seed in all categories. Zinc is the mineral world's own beauty jewel, and pumpkin seeds contain the biggest punch of zinc above all else. Zinc deficiency is linked to both acne and gray hair. As a former acne patient just beginning to gray, pumpkin seeds are a staple in my kitchen.

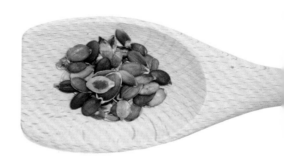

Goji berry

Well, obviously, you'd want a sweet-and-sour antiwrinkle berry in your kitchen pantry. Contains carotenoids (which protect the skin against sun damage), important amino acids, fibers, and antioxidants. Buy only organic.

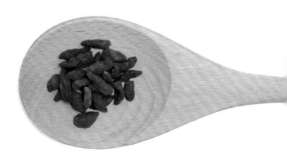

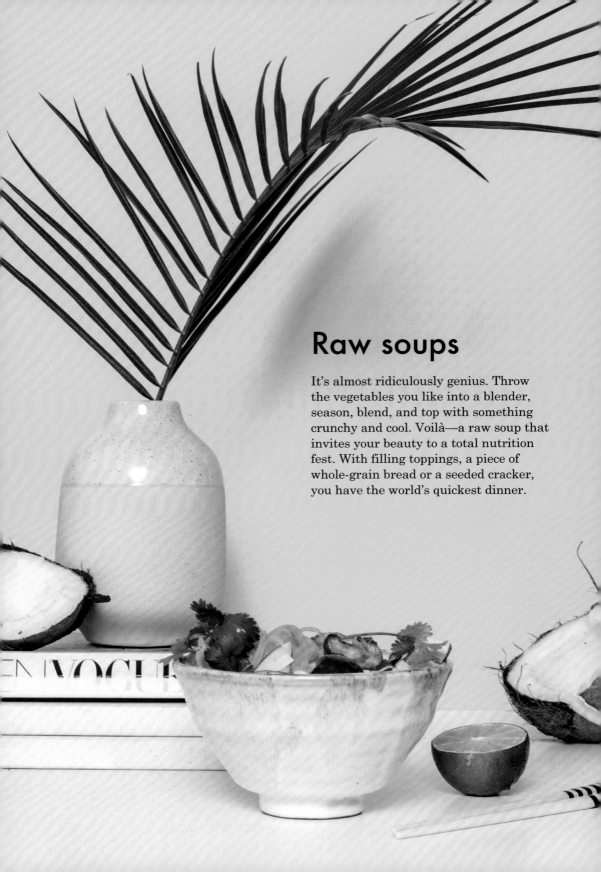

Raw soups

It's almost ridiculously genius. Throw the vegetables you like into a blender, season, blend, and top with something crunchy and cool. Voilà—a raw soup that invites your beauty to a total nutrition fest. With filling toppings, a piece of whole-grain bread or a seeded cracker, you have the world's quickest dinner.

Vegan tom kha with carrot noodles, coconut, and tamari mushrooms

Tom kha gai is a traditional coconut and chicken soup in Thai cuisine. This vegetarian version is almost raw, and stuffed with beauty-boosting vitamins and antioxidants. The most beautiful noodles are carrot noodles made with a spiralizer, but a potato peeler will also do the job. If you want, you can quickly heat the soup in a saucepan, but it should not come to a boil.

2 SERVINGS
CARROT NOODLES
2 carrots

SESAME AND TAMARI-MARINATED MUSHROOMS
10 mushrooms, either white button or shiitake
1 tablespoon sesame oil
1 tablespoon tamari soy sauce

SOUP
2 tomatoes
1 lemongrass stalk
1⅔ cups coconut milk
2–3 tablespoons Thai chili paste
   (I use the brand Santa Maria)
juice of 2 limes
dash of Thai fish sauce, if you're not vegetarian
salt (optional)

TOPPING
cilantro leaves
fresh coconut pieces

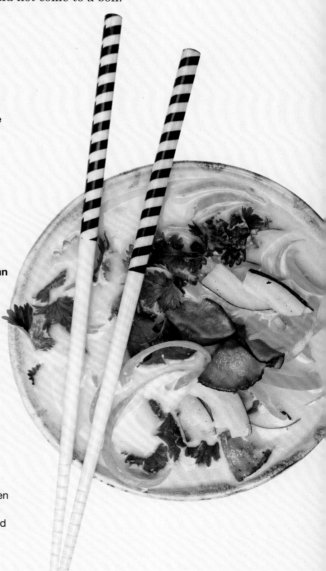

Peel the carrots, then, using a spiralizer, turn them into noodles or shave into thin ribbons with a potato peeler. Set aside.

Cut the mushrooms into decently large pieces. Pour the sesame oil and tamari into a bowl. Massage the mushrooms in the liquid and let marinate for about 15 minutes.

Coarsely chop the tomatoes and lemongrass, then blend with the coconut milk, chili paste, and lime juice until smooth. Season with the fish sauce and salt, if using.

Divide the carrots and mushrooms between 2 bowls. Pour in the soup and top with cilantro and coconut pieces.

Glowpacho

Is there such a thing as a wrinkle moisturizer in liquid form? I believe this recipe fits the bill. It was inspired by the world's finest raw gazpacho at the Flax & Kale restaurant in Barcelona. Let the soup stand in the refrigerator overnight so the flavors come together. Magical!

2 SERVINGS

1 carrot
5 tomatoes
1 red bell pepper
1 cucumber
1 avocado
juice of 1 lemon
2 tablespoons good-quality olive oil
1 tablespoon nutritional yeast flakes
  (found in health-food stores)
1 tablespoon organic vegan bouillon
  powder (not cubes)
1 tablespoon onion powder or granules
1 tablespoon garlic powder
salt and pepper

TOPPINGS
Possibilities include sprouts, finely chopped
  cucumber and tomato, toasted sunflower
  seeds or pumpkin seeds

Peel the carrot. Coarsely chop the carrot, tomatoes, red bell pepper, cucumber, and avocado. Blend the vegetables in a blender until smooth.

Add the lemon juice, olive oil, yeast flakes, bouillon powder, onion powder or granules, and garlic powder. Season with salt and pepper.

Chill the soup, preferably overnight but at least for a few hours, so the flavors can develop.

Sprinkle the soup with your chosen toppings and set out bowls of extra toppings to serve.

BEAUTY BONUS NO. 19

Glowpacho treats you to a super combo of beauty vitamins, antioxidants, minerals, and luster-enhancing fats. Lycopene, which is the red pigment in tomatoes, protects the skin against sun damage and triggers collagen production.

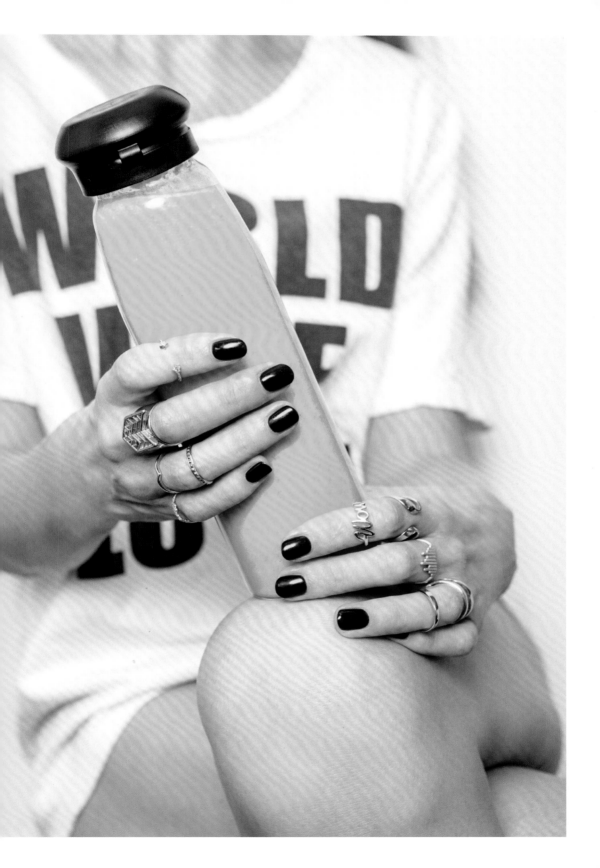

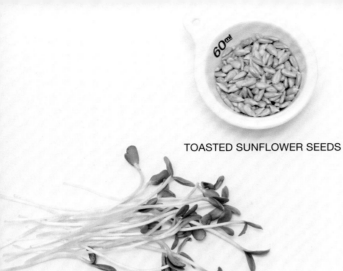

TOASTED SUNFLOWER SEEDS

ALFALFA SROUTS

SUNFLOWER SPROUTS

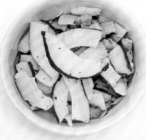

TOASTED COCONUT CHIPS

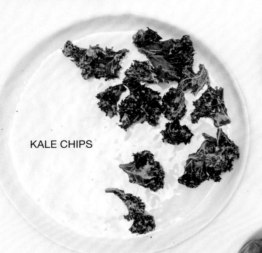

KALE CHIPS

TAMARI-ROASTED ALMONDS

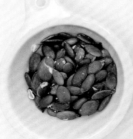

Top your soup!

Crunchy and chewy toppings are the best. These favorites are on constant repeat in my kitchen.

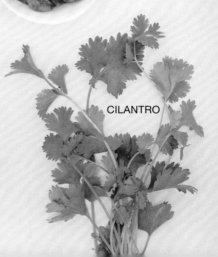

CILANTRO

TOASTED PUMPKIN SEEDS

Greenpacho

During the 1980s and 90s' fatty-food panic, our poor skin was denied the amazing beauty fruit, avocado. This soup is like a green miracle serum for inside your body. I usually sprinkle toasted pumpkin seeds, kale chips, or loads of fresh cilantro on top.

2 SERVINGS
1 cucumber, plus 1 extra, if required
2 avocados
2 large tomatoes
2 cups baby spinach
juice of 1 lemon
1 garlic clove
1 tablespoon good-quality olive oil
1 tablespoon organic vegan bouillon
**   powder (not cubes)**
1 tablespoon onion powder or granules
pinch of chili powder (optional)
salt and pepper

TOPPINGS
possibilities include toasted pumpkin seeds,
**   kale chips, or cilantro leaves**

Coarsely chop the cucumber, avocados, and tomatoes. Blend the chopped ingredients with the spinach, lemon juice, and garlic until smooth, adding water or another cucumber, if necessary. Add the remaining ingredients and season with salt and pepper.

Pour into 2 bowls, and top off each with your chosen toppings.

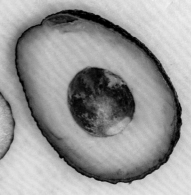

BEAUTY BONUS NO. 20

Avocado offers a bonanza of monounsaturated fats that moisturize the skin from the inside, filling fiber, and important antioxidants, including skin-friendly vitamin E, which protects against UV damage and keeps your skin elastic and glowing.

Slightly more filling glow in a bowl

Beauty bowls, salads, and warm dishes

It's so heavenly to pile up good things in a bowl, mix it all together, and then eat with a spoon (preferably on the couch in front of the television).In this chapter, I avoid giving exact measurements in some recipes. That's because we all love different ingredients, and the nice thing about these bowls is that everyone gets to pile on what they like the most. Each bowl is loaded with beauty foods that inhibit inflammation, support cell renewal, create moisture bombs inside, and give the skin the strength to turn away beauty saboteurs at the door.

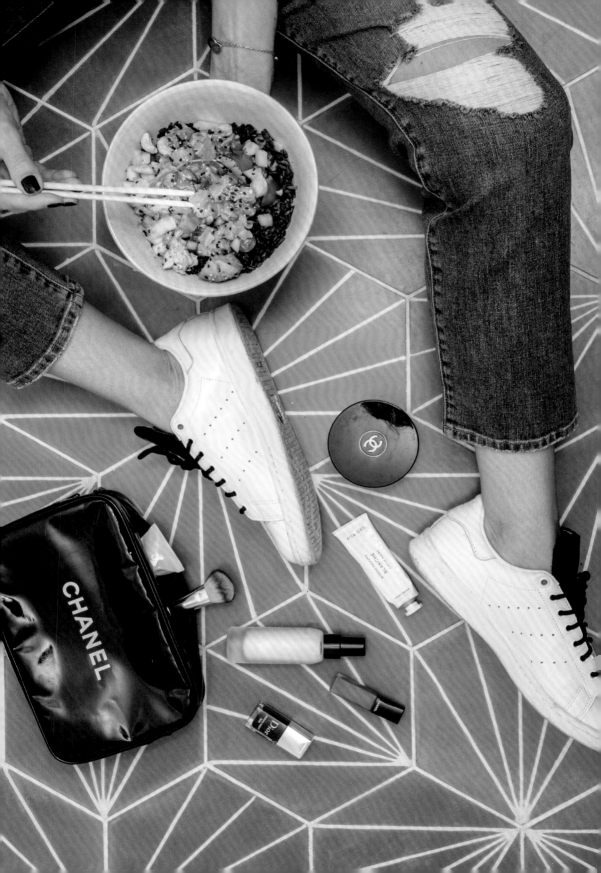

My epic Thai salad

A whole team of beauty-boosting superstars on one and the same plate! There are enough antioxidants to make the nation's collective wrinkles tremble. This salad is also addictively good. My husband sometimes requests this dish on his birthday or when he gets to choose dinner on a cozy Friday night in. I'd like to take the opportunity to point out that my husband, at 41 years old, still gets asked for ID when buying alcohol, which makes this beauty chef mighty proud (and is sometimes worth swearing about, too).

2 SERVING
2 large or 4 small sweet potatoes
½ tablespoon coconut oil
3 tablespoons pumpkin seeds
2 large carrots
1 red bell pepper
2⅓ cups baby spinach
1 avocado
½ lime
2 bunches of cilantro
¾ cup lightly toasted coconut chips
sea salt flakes

CREAMY PEANUT DRESSING WITH LIME AND CHILI
3 tablespoons unsalted peanut butter
½ cup coconut milk
juice of 2 limes
1 tablespoon Thai red curry paste
pinch of sea salt flakes

Preheat the oven to 400°F. Scrub the sweet potatoes, then cut into small chunks and put into a roasting pan lined with parchment paper. Gently melt the coconut oil in a small saucepan or in a microwave. Coat the potatoes in the melted oil and sprinkle with a generous pinch of salt. Roast in the middle of the oven for about 30 minutes, until golden and crispy. Remove from the oven and let cool.

Blend together all the dressing ingredients with a handheld blender, adding a little water if it is too thick, then set aside.

Toast the pumpkin seeds with a pinch of salt in a dry skillet over medium heat until lightly golden. Transfer immediately to a plate and let cool.

Peel the carrots, then cut them and the red bell pepper into thin shreds using a sharp knife or mandoline. Put into a bowl with the baby spinach. Add the halved avocado, sweet potatoes, lime, and generous amounts of cilantro, then sprinkle with the toasted pumpkin seeds and the coconut chips. Top with the creamy peanut dressing.

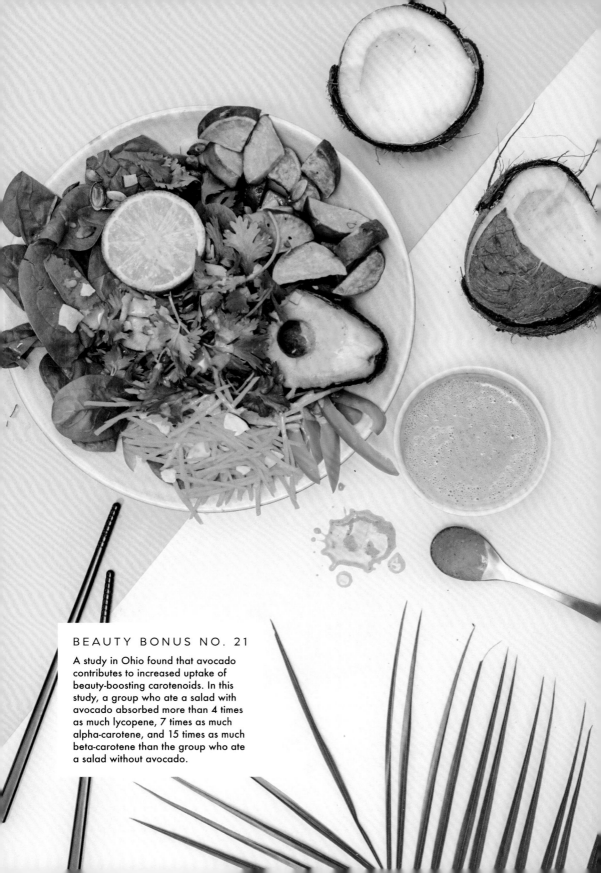

BEAUTY BONUS NO. 21

A study in Ohio found that avocado contributes to increased uptake of beauty-boosting carotenoids. In this study, a group who ate a salad with avocado absorbed more than 4 times as much lycopene, 7 times as much alpha-carotene, and 15 times as much beta-carotene than the group who ate a salad without avocado.

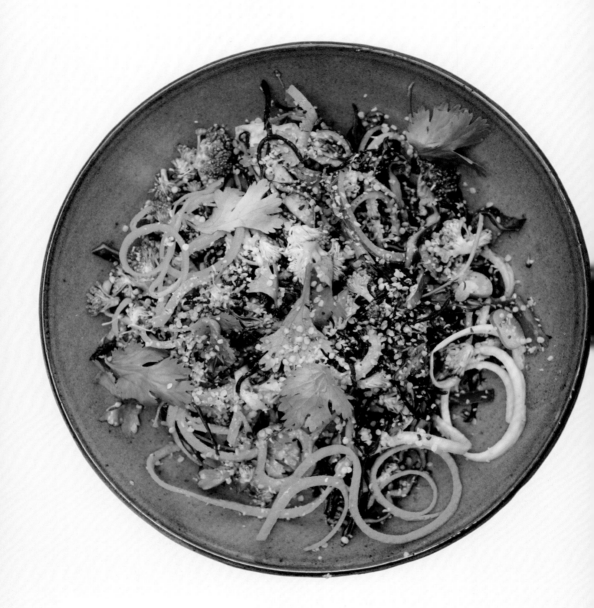

BEAUTY BONUS NO. 22

This is a bowl of pure rocket fuel.
Colorful mixed vegetables provide
a perfect palette of antioxidants,
phytonutrients, and fiber. The
seaweed protects the skin and
gives hair a shiny boost.

Asiatic superbowl with arame and hemp topping

Here, I skip exact measurements. Add in what you like best and have at home. I use the same dressing as the Thai salad on page 62, but if you're feeling lazy, mix together a splash of tamari soy sauce, lime, and sesame oil and use that.

Creamy Peanut Dressing with Lime and Chili
(see page 62)
red cabbage
red onion
broccoli
carrots
zucchini
dried arame seaweed
cilantro leaves
shelled hemp seeds

Make the dressing following the directions on page 62 and put into the refrigerator. Finely shred the red cabbage and red onion. Chop the broccoli into small florets. Peel the carrots. Using a spiralizer, turn the carrots and zucchini into noodles.

Soak the arame according to the package directions, then drain.

Put the prepared vegetables into a bowl. Pour the dressing over them and stir everything thoroughly so that the vegetables soften and become flavorful. Top with the arame, cilantro leaves, and hemp seeds.

TIP!
You can easily make vegetable noodles yourself with a spiralizer. Mine cost less than 15 dollars in a typical kitchenware store. You can also make long, thin ribbons with the help of a potato peeler, but it's a little more difficult.

Beluga, tomato, and parsley salad with lemon dressing

We spend every summer in Juan-les-Pins on the French Riviera, and life is more or less about sitting on the balcony and eating salad made from the day's finds at the market and drinking pale rosé wine. Dinner isn't served until nine in the evening, and the balcony fills with the powdery scent of French skincare brand Nuxe's After-Sun product (my favorite).

2 SERVINGS
½–¾ cup dried black beluga lentils or
   French green lentils
several pinches of dried thyme, oregano,
   and/or rosemary (if you have a herbes de
   Provence blend, that would be great) or
   organic vegan bouillon powder
handful of small vine-ripened tomatoes
   (tomatoes taste best when ripened on
   the vine)
1 red bell pepper
½ red onion
a small bunch of parsley
1 avocado
a piece of watermelon
a handful of walnuts
salt and pepper

LEMON AND HONEY DRESSING
finely grated zest and juice of 1 lemon
½ cup olive oil
2 teaspoons honey
salt and pepper

Cook the lentils according to the package directions, adding the dried herbs or bouillon powder to the cooking water. Drain, if necessary, then let cool completely.

For the dressing, mix the lemon juice and zest with the olive oil, honey, and salt and pepper. Set aside.

Finely chop the tomatoes, red bell pepper, onion, and parsley, then put into a large bowl and add the lentils.

Cube the avocado and watermelon, then add to the salad. Add the coarsely chopped walnuts, a little salt and pepper, and the dressing and toss together.

TIP!
When barbecuing for guests, this chic salad is the perfect accompaniment to grilled salmon or halloumi.

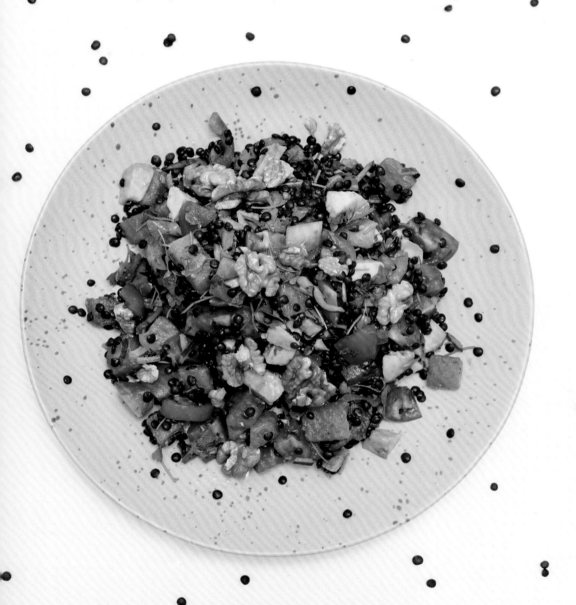

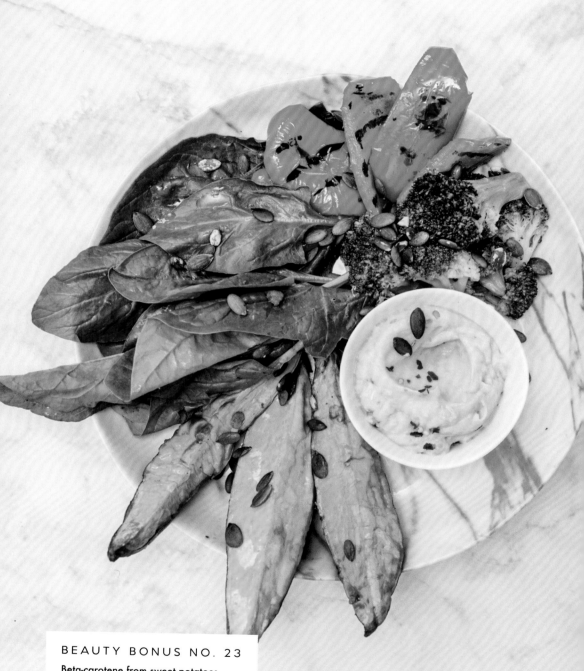

BEAUTY BONUS NO. 23

Beta-carotene from sweet potatoes, vitamin E from avocados, vitamin K from spinach and broccoli, and pimple-fighting zinc from pumpkin seeds make this a staple in the beauty kitchen.

Roasted sweet potatoes with avocado fluff

This is a beauty food variation on French fries with Béarnaise sauce. If you like, you can add a sprinkle of seaweed salt instead of sea salt flakes to create an incredible umami flavor (the fifth basic flavor—a deep savoriness), which can be hard to produce in vegetarian food. This would also provide bonus beauty points, thanks to the metabolic-boosting iodine in the seaweed.

2 SERVINGS
2 sweet potatoes
1 red bell pepper
1 tablespoon coconut oil
1 cup broccoli florets
⅓ cup pumpkin seeds
2⅓ cups baby spinach
balsamic vinegar (optional)
sea salt flakes

AVOCADO FLUFF
2 avocados
juice of 1 lemon
2 garlic cloves
**pinch of smoked paprika powder
  or chili flakes**
salt and pepper

Blend together all the avocado fluff ingredients with a handheld blender, season with salt and pepper, and put into the refrigerator.

Preheat the oven to 400°F. Peel the sweet potatoes, then slice into thin wedges. Slice the red bell pepper into chunks.

Gently melt the coconut oil in a small saucepan or in a microwave. Coat the prepared sweet potatoes, red bell pepper, and broccoli florets with the melted oil and sprinkle with sea salt flakes.

Put the vegetables into a roasting pan lined with parchment paper and roast in the middle of the oven. After 20 minutes, increase the temperature to 425°F and bake for another 10 minutes, until the edges of the vegetables are crispy. You may need to pluck out the broccoli a little sooner, and perhaps even the red bell pepper, so keep an eye on things. Toss the pumpkin seeds over the vegetables 5 minutes before the end of the cooking time, so that they have time to get some color.

Let the vegetables cool slightly, then serve with the avocado fluff and baby spinach. A drop of balsamic vinegar on the spinach is delicious.

Forever young sweet-and-sour salad with lemon and tahini dressing

Choose a really sour green apple, such as Granny Smith, for this salad.

2 SERVINGS
⅔ cup frozen shelled edamame (soybeans)
½ red cabbage
juice of 2 limes
1 tablespoon sesame oil
1 red bell pepper
1 yellow bell pepper
1 apple
2 bunches of cilantro
2 bunches of mint

LEMON AND TAHINI DRESSING
1-inch piece of fresh ginger
3 tablespoons tahini
3 tablespoons olive oil
finely grated zest and juice of 1 large lemon
1 tablespoon yacon syrup (coconut nectar or maple syrup also work)
salt

TOPPING
a few spoonfuls of sunflower seeds
seeds of 1 pomegranate
sea salt flakes

Boil the edamame for about 2 minutes. Refresh in cold water, then drain and set aside.

To make the dressing, peel and grate the ginger, then blend with the tahini, olive oil, lemon juice, lemon zest, and syrup using a handheld blender. Season with salt and set aside.

Shred the red cabbage. Massage with the lime juice, sesame oil, and a little salt until it softens. Slice the bell peppers and apple into matchsticks. Stir together the bell peppers, apple, cabbage, edamame, and dressing, then add the cilantro and mint leaves.

Toast the sunflower seeds with a little salt in a dry skillet over medium heat. Set aside to cool.

Top with the toasted sunflower seeds, pomegranate seeds, and a few flakes of sea salt.

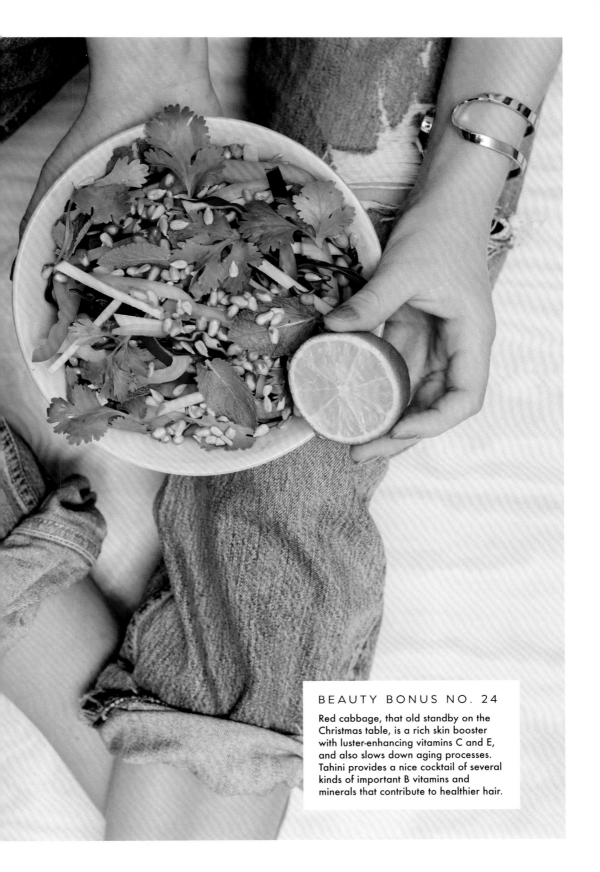

BEAUTY BONUS NO. 24

Red cabbage, that old standby on the Christmas table, is a rich skin booster with luster-enhancing vitamins C and E, and also slows down aging processes. Tahini provides a nice cocktail of several kinds of important B vitamins and minerals that contribute to healthier hair.

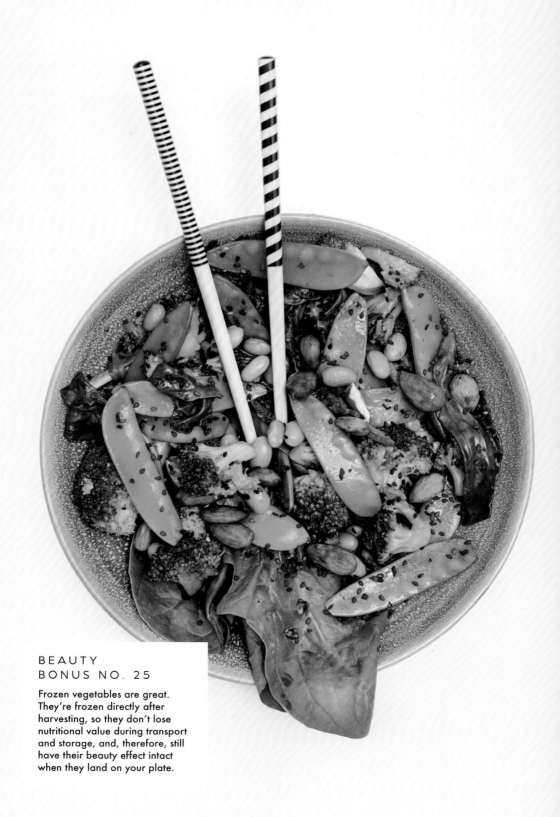

BEAUTY
BONUS NO. 25

Frozen vegetables are great.
They're frozen directly after
harvesting, so they don't lose
nutritional value during transport
and storage, and, therefore, still
have their beauty effect intact
when they land on your plate.

Easy Monday wok with supergreens, tamari, and beauty topping

This is my standby Monday dish. It (a.) compensates for the weekend's nonbeauty-compatible debauchery and (b.) requires zero effort, taking less than 5 minutes to go from the freezer to your mouth. Yes, you read that correctly. Here, the whole beauty troupe, except for the toppings and spinach leaves, comes from the freezer. Choose frozen vegetables of good quality, preferably early produce if available. Equal-size, tender broccoli florets with many crowns on them and little stem are the best. To make the dish more filling, you can add diced tofu or serve with a piece of salmon.

2 SERVINGS

1 tablespoon coconut oil
3 cups frozen broccoli
⅔ cup frozen sugar snap peas
⅔ cup frozen shelled edamame (soybeans)
1 garlic clove
2–3 tablespoons tamari soy sauce
2 cups baby spinach
1 tablespoon sesame oil

TOPPING
black sesame seeds
tamari-roasted almonds (available
  in well-stocked health-food stores
  and grocery stores)

Heat the coconut oil in a skillet or wok. Add the broccoli, sugar snap peas, edamame, and crushed garlic and stir-fry over high heat for about 3 minutes, or until everything is heated through. Stir in the tamari and reduce the heat. Mix in the spinach and turn off the heat.

Transfer to a bowl, drizzle with the sesame oil, and top off with sesame seeds and almonds.

Skin-tox superbowl with sesame salmon with mango and lime salsa

This, my friends, is a total orgy of first-class beauty food. Paired with ice-cold white wine, it's also luxurious enough to serve at a party. Any sashimi-grade salmon will work a charm for this.

2 SERVINGS
10½ oz sashimi-grade salmon
pinch of sea salt flakes
¼ cup black and white sesame seeds,
  plus extra to serve
1⅓ cups frozen shelled edamame (soybeans)
1 cucumber
2–3 scallions
2⅓ cups baby spinach or other leafy greens
a sprig of cilantro

CARIBBEAN MANGO AND LIME SALSA
1 fresh mango or 1½ cups frozen and
  defrosted mango chunks
juice and finely grated zest of 1 lime
½ tablespoon finely grated fresh ginger
½ red chili
salt

To make the salsa, blend the mango flesh, lime juice, and ginger until smooth. Finely chop the chili and stir in along with the lime zest. Season with salt and put into the refrigerator.

Preheat the oven to 400°F. Slice the salmon into large pieces. Mix the salt flakes and sesame seeds on a plate, then coat the salmon pieces with the mixture. Put into a baking dish and bake in the middle of the oven for 6–8 minutes, depending on the size of the salmon pieces, until just cooked through (sashimi-grade salmon is best when a little raw in the middle, so don't overbake it).

Meanwhile, boil the edamame for about 2 minutes. Refresh in cold water, then drain. Using a potato peeler, slice the cucumber into long ribbons. Chop the scallions into small pieces. Put the spinach or other greens into a bowl with the edamame, scallions, salmon, and cucumber.

Serve with the mango and lime salsa, cilantro sprig, and some extra sesame seeds.

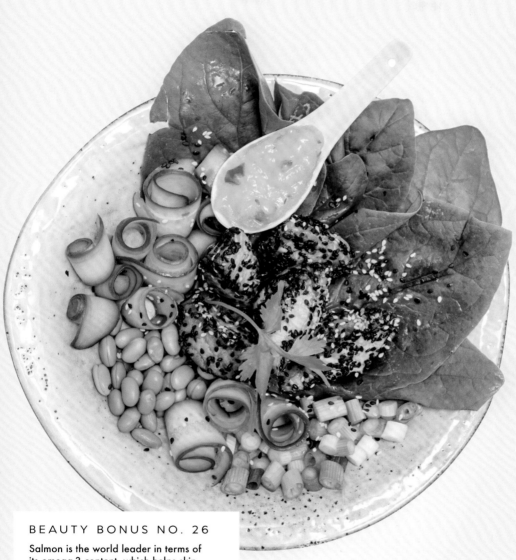

BEAUTY BONUS NO. 26

Salmon is the world leader in terms of
its omega-3 content, which helps skin
stay smooth, lustrous, and even toned.
The pink pigment astaxanthin is a true
superantioxidant. Although farmed salmon
contains less omega-3 than those caught
in the wild, I prefer it because it doesn't
contain as many potential pollutants.
Please choose sustainable salmon.

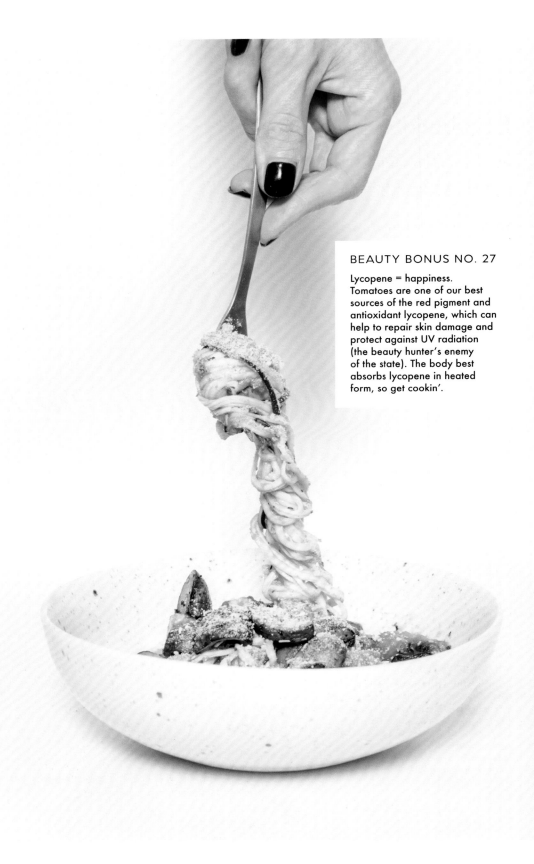

BEAUTY BONUS NO. 27

Lycopene = happiness. Tomatoes are one of our best sources of the red pigment and antioxidant lycopene, which can help to repair skin damage and protect against UV radiation (the beauty hunter's enemy of the state). The body best absorbs lycopene in heated form, so get cookin'.

Skin-lovin' spaghetti marinara with garlic-fried mushrooms and pumpkin "parmesan"

The world's most skin-friendly pasta dish, topped with pumpkin "parmesan" that will make your hair stand on end. Nutritional yeast flakes have the most unsexy name in the food pantry, but they have a unique umami cheese flavor and the B-vitamin content is fantastic for hair and nails. Vegans often lack B_{12}, so nutritional yeast should be a constant companion. Mix the flakes with zinc-rich pumpkin seeds for a raw "parmesan" that is totally addictive. Store what's left over in a tightly sealed glass jar in a cool, dark place.

2 SERVINGS
1 large zucchini

MARINARA SAUCE
1 small white onion
2 garlic cloves
1 tablespoon olive oil
1 (14½-oz) can diced tomatoes
1 tablespoon organic vegan bouillon powder (not cubes)
2 teaspoons honey
2 teaspoons dried thyme
10 cherry tomatoes

GARLIC-FRIED MUSHROOMS
8 oz mushrooms (cremini mushrooms work well)
½ tablespoon olive oil
2–3 garlic cloves
salt and pepper

PUMPKIN "PARMESAN"
¾ cup pumpkin seeds
1½ cups nutritional yeast flakes (found in health-food stores)
1 teaspoon garlic powder (optional)
1 teaspoon sea salt flakes

Combine the pumpkin "parmesan" ingredients in a food processor until they are evenly distributed. Scrape the mixture from the edges as necessary, but don't process it too long. You want a crumblike texture, not butter.

For the garlic-fried mushrooms, slice the mushrooms into quarters. Heat the olive oil in a skillet. Add the mushrooms and crushed garlic. Sauté until golden, then season with salt and pepper. Set aside.

For the sauce, finely chop the onion and garlic. Heat the olive oil in a deep saucepan. Sauté the onion over medium heat until translucent, about 5 minutes. Add the garlic and cook, stirring, for a few minutes. Pour in the diced tomatoes and bouillon powder and cook until the sauce begins to bubble. Reduce the heat, cover, and let simmer for at least 20 minutes—the longer the better.

Meanwhile, using a spiralizer, turn the zucchini into spaghetti or shave into long, thin ribbons with a potato peeler.

Season the tomato sauce with the honey, thyme, and salt and pepper. Halve the cherry tomatoes and stir into the sauce. Add the zucchini "spaghetti" and stir everything until well combined. Finally, add the mushrooms. Serve sprinkled with the pumpkin "parmesan."

Zesty (almost raw) vegan pad thai

Kelp (seaweed) noodles can be long, so cut them into shorter, bite-size pieces. In this dish, I like their crispness, but shirataki noodles work excellently, if you prefer a softer consistency.

2 SERVINGS
1 zucchini
1 peeled carrot
¼ red cabbage
10½ oz kelp (seaweed) noodles

PAD THAI DRESSING
3 tablespoons peanut butter
½ cup coconut milk
juice of 2 limes
1 garlic clove, crushed
1 tablespoon Thai red curry paste
pinch of sea salt flakes

TO SERVE
2 large bunches of cilantro
a handful of unsalted roasted peanuts
2 limes
2 scallions (optional)

Mix together all the dressing ingredients, then set aside.

Using a spiralizer, turn the zucchini and carrot into noodles, or shave into thin ribbons with a potato peeler. Finely shred the red cabbage. Soak the kelp noodles according to the package directions, then drain.

Put the vegetables and the well-drained noodles into a large bowl along with the dressing. Stir until everything is well combined. Serve with plenty of cilantro, the peanuts, lime wedges, and finely sliced scallions, if you want.

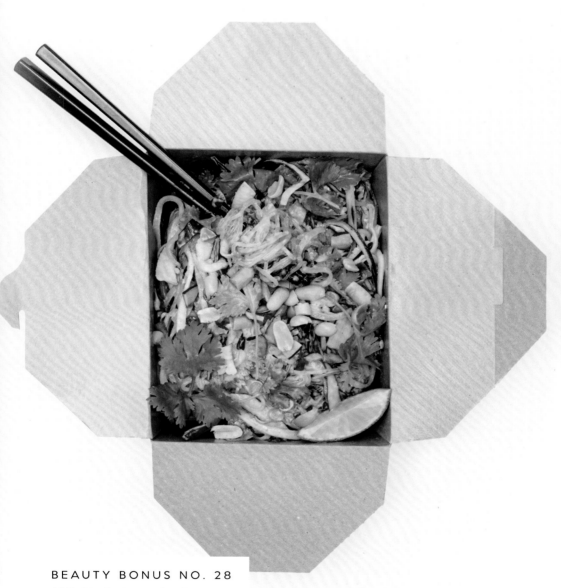

BEAUTY BONUS NO. 28

All kindds of onions, and garlic, too,
are beauty kitchen heroes. Cleansing,
anti-inflammatory effects build defenses
against both pimples and fine lines,
while flavonoids produce sky-high
antioxidant activity.

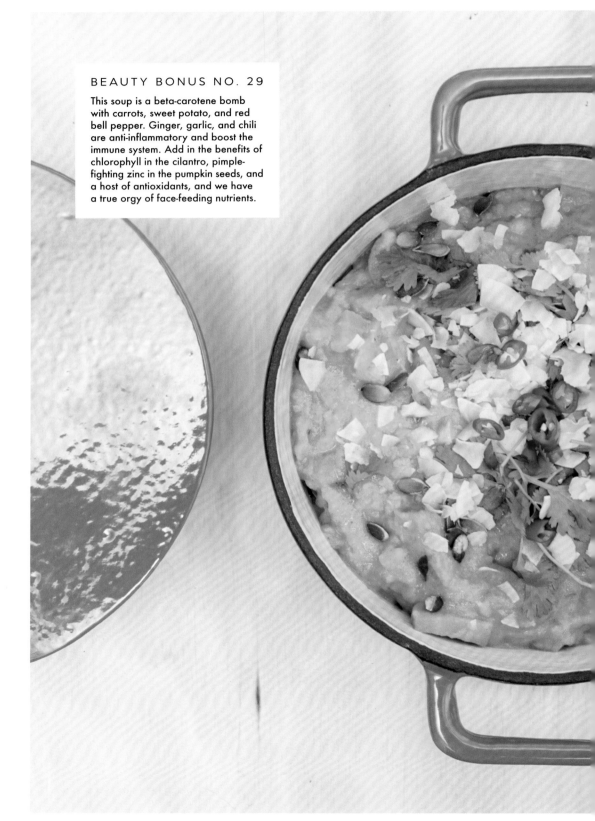

BEAUTY BONUS NO. 29

This soup is a beta-carotene bomb
with carrots, sweet potato, and red
bell pepper. Ginger, garlic, and chili
are anti-inflammatory and boost the
immune system. Add in the benefits of
chlorophyll in the cilantro, pimple-
fighting zinc in the pumpkin seeds, and
a host of antioxidants, and we have
a true orgy of face-feeding nutrients.

Thai carrot and sweet potato soup (aka The warming gatekeeper for man flu and wrinkles)

Face feeders, sun worshippers, and winter cold sufferers, this one is for you! It's also the perfect soup to make for someone near and dear with a cold coming on. Anything that can stop man flu from entering the household earns my eternal love. The soup is spicy and might make you sniffle a little over the bowl. I love a touch of chili, but there have been times when I've eaten dishes in Thai restaurants in Asia that were so strong I thought I was going deaf, and felt so dizzy that I had to be taken home by taxi.

2–3 SERVINGS

3 shallots or 1 yellow onion
3 large garlic cloves
2-inch piece of fresh ginger
2 tablespoons coconut oil
1–3 tablespoons Thai red curry paste,
   to taste
1 large sweet potato
4–5 large carrots
1 red bell pepper
¾ cup dried red lentils
1 tablespoon organic vegan bouillon powder
2½ cups water
1⅔ cups coconut milk
about 6 dried kaffir lime leaves
juice of 1 lime
a few drops of Thai fish sauce (optional)

TOPPINGS
2 bunches of cilantro
toasted pumpkin seeds
toasted coconut chips
1 red chili

Peel and finely chop the shallots or onion and the garlic. Peel and shred the ginger. Heat the coconut oil in a large saucepan and cook the shallots or onion over medium heat for about 4 minutes, until soft. Add the garlic and cook for another minute. Add the ginger and curry paste and reduce the heat. Think low 'n' slow—letting everything revel over low heat for a while deepens the delicious flavors.

Peel the sweet potato and carrots. Cut them and the red bell pepper into pieces. Increase the heat and put the vegetables into the saucepan. Stir thoroughly so the flavors infuse everything, then let sputter for a few minutes. Pour in the lentils (optionally rinsed in a colander), sprinkle with the bouillon powder, and stir in the measured water. Bring to a boil, then reduce the heat and mix in the coconut milk and lime leaves. Simmer for at least 25 minutes, adding more water if necessary, until the carrots and sweet potato are soft.

Remove from heat, pick out the lime leaves and blend the soup with a handheld blender, just enough to leave some chunky pieces. Stir in the lime juice and a few drops of fish sauce, if using, to get that umami flavor.

Sprinkle with the coarsely chopped cilantro, the pumpkin seeds, the coconut chips, and the sliced red chili. The toppings can, of course, vary, depending on what you have at home.

TIP!
Lime leaves lend a deep lime flavor. Don't forget to pluck them out before you blend the soup. If you can't find lime leaves, don't worry. Just squeeze in a little extra lime juice instead to add the same flavor.

Follow the *hara hachi bu* rule and eat until you're 80 percent full. (Note! I've never had much luck following this rule.)

Eat food in its original or its least prepared form as much as possible. Simplicity is best.

Eating with *hashi* (chopsticks) means we eat more slowly and the stomach can keep up with the tempo. Glowing skin begins in the stomach, ladies!

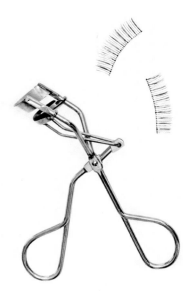

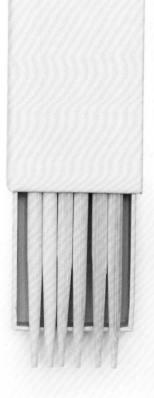

My Japanese beauty kitchen

Miso, soba, and Japanese soul food

In January 2007, I moved to Tokyo and life would never be the same again. Neither would my skin, but I didn't know that then. When I landed at Tokyo airport, I had no idea that, four years later, I would look at edamame (soybeans) and miso as part of my skincare routine, find joy in covering my face in cloths soaked in serum and snail slime (this was long before face masks were discovered in the rest of the world), or stand under a UV-protective umbrella during the summer.

Ever since the time of the geishas, skin has been a source of pride for Japanese women. I was completely dazzled by the porcelain cheeks of Japanese people, which were in stark contrast to the tanned and slightly dragonlike Botox ideal of the Western world.

In the fashionable neighborhood of the city, there were several beauty food cafés where each dish was described by its beauty benefits, and I became a regular at an *izakaya* Japanese restaurant that had a special cocktail menu for skin beauty. I even drank a nighttime drink that promised to preserve my youth (which I also severely threatened with cigarettes and cheap wine at karaoke bars).

My whole approach to food changed in Japan. Instead of removing things from a Western diet, I added things that strengthened my body and, it soon seemed, my personal display window—my skin and hair. I discovered that by adding a lot of good stuff to my daily menu, less delicious stuff naturally began to disappoint.

Obviously, it takes more than a single tofu steak to turn tired skin into tight skin, smooth as a peach, but by eating organic vegetables, fish, miso, algae, and fresh fruit, I promise that you, like me, will soon see beautiful skin in the mirror. Combine that with rigorous UV protection and you'll have a wonderful future. The snail slime is optional.

Japanese beauty food

ALGAE
Algae are a skin-boosting miracle, providing all the essential amino acids we need, plus minerals and antioxidants that help the skin repair itself and protect against aging. Some of my favorites are arame, hijiki, dulse, nori, and wakame. (Note: If you're pregnant, eat only small amounts of hijiki, because some products have been found to contain low levels of arsenic.)

BROWN RICE
Unpolished, short-grain brown rice (genmai) has a high fiber content and a lot of the B vitamins and minerals that contribute to smooth skin, beautiful hair and strong nails. It also contains ceramides, a type of fat that helps create a moisturized and well-functioning skin barrier. As you'll see, I use brown rice freely in everything from salads to sushi.

EDAMAME
These green soybeans are rich in phytochemical isoflavones that can slow down the degradation of collagen, the protein that makes the skin firm and smooth. In a U.S. study, it was noted that mice fed with isoflavones managed UV exposure better and had smoother skin than their friends not fed isoflavones.

FATTY FISH
Omega-3 fatty acid does wonders for the skin, especially dry skin, and has anti-inflammatory properties. Salmon and mackerel are favorite sources. Salmon also contains the pink pigment astaxanthin, a superstar antioxidant from the carotenoid group that inhibits free radical damage. Eat fatty fish three times a week to turn up the glow to the max.

MISO
Fermented soybean paste is one of Japan's most important staple ingredients. It's bubbling with anti-inflammatory and immune-boosting properties, and it strengthens the good bacterial flora in the stomach. I can't stress this more—happy stomachs are the alpha and omega of happy skin. In addition to soup, miso is amazingly delicious in marinades, dressings, and vegetable dips. In Japan, you can find an unbelievable number of miso varieties—from sweet white to musty, dark red. Sometimes rice or oats are added to the fermentation process. Buy unpasteurized miso in which the heat-sensitive enzymes are intact. Boiling destroys both the taste of the miso and the enzymes. Handle this Japanese "gold" carefully and it will reward you with a glow, inside and out.

NATTO
A pressed mass of fermented soybeans, natto is made in Japan for its many health and beauty properties. However, natto is a real stink bomb, but this is quickly forgiven by beauty foodies because of its high content of the nutrient pyrroloquinoline quinone (PQQ), which, according to studies, appears to protect the cells' own small energy engines, mitochondria, and also contributes to keeping them working in aging cells. A beauty food for the truly dedicated.

SESAME SEEDS
These beautiful seeds contain good minerals, fatty acids, and vitamin E, which can protect against free radicals. Unhulled sesame seeds have more nutrition than hulled, but they must be crushed before eating in order for the nutrition to be released.

SHIITAKE
This fluttering little mushroom works as an anti-inflammatory and protects our DNA from free-radical damage. In some studies, there's been a connection between shiitake and decreased acne. Available both dried and fresh, for different uses.

SOBA
Known as buckwheat in English, although it's not a wheat but a herb, soba contains plenty of amino acids, the B vitamins, fiber, and antioxidants. Soba noodles are excellent both cold and hot.

TOFU
Without exception, my Japanese friends praise tofu as one of the secrets behind their smooth skin. Tofu is full of protein and isoflavones, which prevent collagen degradation and make for a resilient, firm skin. In addition to cooking, it's also used in pastries, such as tofu tiramisu and tofu cheesecake.

Hijiki kinpira—soy and sesame sautéed carrots with hijiki

Kinpira means "sauté and simmer," and the technique is used for a range of creative vegetable side dishes. In Japan, kinpira is a given element in the bento box. I was especially fond of kinpira with carrot and hijiki (a type of algae, see page 84), which gives a dramatic blackness and a lot of beauty minerals. The carrots are loaded with skin-loving beta-carotene, and the sesame seeds with calcium. Serve as a side or as a main dish in a large bowl of short-grain brown rice, lightly fried tofu, edamame (soybeans), and greens.

2 SERVINGS (OR 4 SERVED AS A SIDE DISH)
2¾ oz dried hijiki
3 small or 2 large peeled carrots
1 tablespoon sesame oil
3 tablespoons shoyu or Japanese soy sauce
2 tablespoons mirin
1 cup dashi (see page 87) or water

TO GARNISH
2 tablespoons unhulled white sesame seeds

Rinse the hijiki, then soak in cold water for about 30 minutes. Meanwhile, cut the carrots into superthin sticks about 2¾ inches long.

Drain the hijiki. Heat the sesame oil in a deep skillet over medium heat. Add the carrots and well-drained hijiki and stir so that everything is coated in the oil. Sauté until everything is soft, about 4 minutes. Pour in the shoyu or soy sauce, mirin, and dashi or water. Reduce the heat to low and simmer for about 20 minutes, until all the liquid has evaporated.

Meanwhile, toast the sesame seeds in a dry skillet until golden. Transfer immediately to a plate, because they burn easily. Put the hijiki kinpira into a bowl and let cool for a few minutes. Sprinkle with the toasted sesame seeds and enjoy.

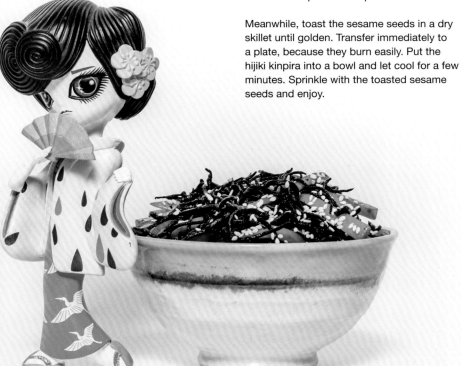

Tofu salad with Mia-san's ginger-spiked sesame and peanut dressing

My Tokyo friend Mia makes a terrific dressing with toasted sesame seeds. It's creamy, a little spicy, and dizzyingly good. You will have (maybe) some leftover dressing, which will last for up to a week in an airtight container in the refrigerator.

2 SERVINGS
9 oz firm tofu
2 carrots
3⅓ cups mixed greens (preferably including a peppery variety, such as arugula)

SESAME AND PEANUT DRESSING
½ cup white sesame seeds
½ red chili (optional)
¼ cup unsalted peanut butter
2 garlic cloves, crushed (optional)
1 tablespoon grated fresh ginger
5 tablespoons shoyu or Japanese soy sauce
2 tablespoons rice vinegar
½ tablespoon coconut nectar or coconut sugar
1–2 tablespoons water (warm water if using coconut sugar, so that it loosens up)

TO GARNISH
1 tablespoon black sesame seeds

Press the tofu to make it firmer: Wrap the tofu block in double-layered paper towels. Put it onto a plate, then place another plate on top (preferably adding a weight on top of that). Let stand for about 30 minutes.

Meanwhile, make the dressing. Toast the white sesame seeds in a dry skillet over medium heat until golden. Transfer immediately to a plate and let cool. Chop the chilli, if using. Blend the toasted sesame seeds and chili with the other ingredients, adding small amounts of the measured water at a time so that the dressing doesn't become too thin. Mix to a perfectly smooth, creamy dressing.

Cut the tofu into cubes. Peel the carrots, then cut them into long, thin ribbons with a potato peeler.

Put the mixed greens, carrots, and tofu into a bowl, drizzle with the dressing, and sprinkle with the black sesame seeds.

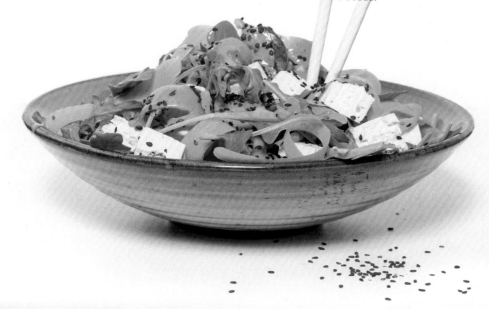

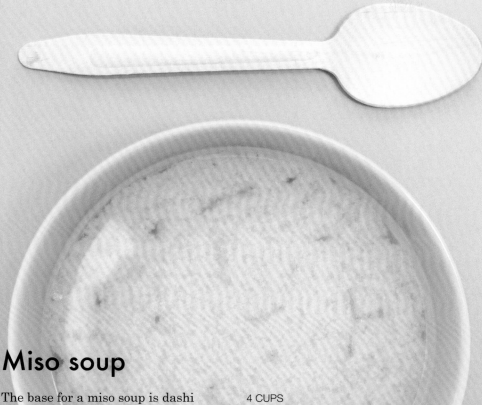

Miso soup

The base for a miso soup is dashi (broth) and miso paste. In Japan, dashi often contains flakes of smoked and dried bonito fish, but this variant—kombu dashi—is made of only kombu seaweed, which makes it vegan-friendly and crazy simple to make. White miso is mild, while red is musty and earthy. An important thing: Never let miso soup boil—it destroys the flavor and the beauty-boosting bacteria and enzymes, which defeats the whole point.

4 CUPS
¾ oz dried kombu seaweed
4 cups water
⅓ cup miso paste

To make the dashi, don't rinse the kombu, which reduces its umami flavor. Make a few cuts in the sheet, but keeping the sheet in one piece. Put it into a bowl and pour over the measured water. Let soak in the refrigerator for 10 hours. Remove the kombu sheet. Your kombu dashi is ready.

Bring the dashi to a boil in a saucepan. Remove from the heat and pour into a heatproof bowl. Stir the miso paste into the dashi until it is completely dissolved. Pour back into the saucepan and warm over low heat.

GOOD STUFF TO PUT IN THE MISO SOUP
wakame seaweed, presoaked for 5 minutes
diced tofu
sliced scallions

Sparkling green miso soup

This soup is an act of charity for the body, soul, and beauty. It is inspired by
a recipe for Chinese medicinal soup in a cookbook I bought in Bali many years
ago, and, since then, I've free-styled it with Asian flavors such as ginger, sesame,
miso, chilli, shiitake, and cilantro. You can use either miso paste or instant
miso soup.

2 SERVINGS

1 chili
3 garlic cloves
2-inch piece of fresh ginger
3½ oz fresh shiitake mushrooms
3½ oz frozen artichokes
1 tablespoon coconut oil
2 cups broccoli florets
1½ tablespoons tamari soy sauce, plus extra
   to serve
1 teaspoon sesame oil, plus extra to serve
3⅓ cups water
¾ cup frozen shelled edamame (soybeans)
2 (⅓-oz) envelopes instant miso soup or
   3 tablespoons white miso paste
7 oz shirataki noodles (soft noodles
   made of konjac root, aka fitness noodles)

TOPPING
2 bunches of cilantro
sunflower sprouts
scallion
furikake (see recipe opposite) or
   toasted sesame seeds

Finely chop the chili, garlic, and peeled ginger.
Slice the mushrooms. Cut the artichokes in half.

Heat the coconut oil in a saucepan. Add the
garlic, ginger, and chili. Sauté over low heat
for about 3 minutes, stirring constantly. Add
the mushrooms, increase the heat, and cook,
stirring. Add the artichokes and broccoli. Pour
in the tamari and bubble for about 1 minute,
until evaporated. Set aside, drizzle with the
sesame oil, and stir.

Bring the measured water to a boil in a
saucepan. Add the edamame (soybeans),
reduce the heat, and cook for 1 minute, then stir
in the instant miso soup or miso paste (the water
must not boil). Rinse the shirataki noodles.

Divide the noodles and fried vegetables between
2 bowls. Pour over the miso and edamame
broth. Top with loads of cilantro, sunflower
sprouts, sliced scallion, and furikake or sesame
seeds. Set out extra sesame oil, tamari, and
furikake and add to taste.

Make your own furikake

Furikake is a mixture of toasted sesame seeds, nori seaweed, and your own choice of seasonings—for example, shiso cress. My variation gives a royal beauty boost, is supereasy to make, and works wonderfully as a topping for rice, salad, soup, or salmon.

ABOUT 2 CUPS
⅔ cup black sesame seeds
⅔ cup white sesame seeds
tiny pinch of sea salt flakes
3 sheets of roasted nori (sushi sheets)

Lightly toast the sesame seeds in a dry skillet over medium heat until they start popping. Pour into a bowl, lightly salt (be sparing, because the seaweed also contains salt), and stir. Cut the nori sheets into small pieces with clean kitchen scissors and stir into the toasted mixture. I like the nori really small, but that's a minor thing—if you like long, fancy strips, of course, it's just as good. Transfer to a glass jar, seal, and store in a cool, dark place.

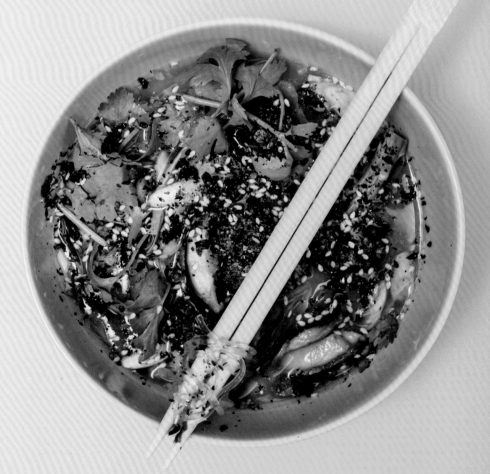

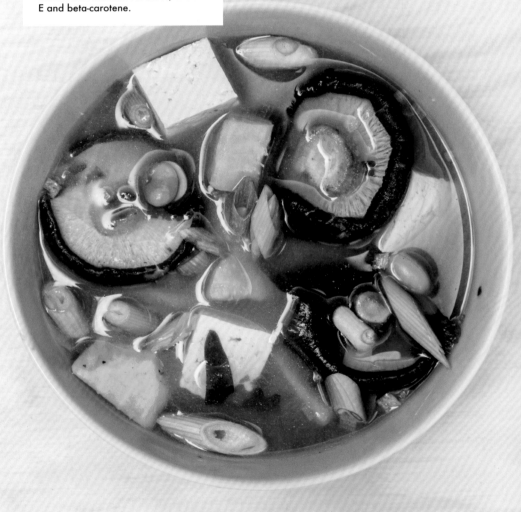

Miso soup with mushroom, sweet potato, and tofu

This soup warms frozen souls and fills the body with beauty love deluxe. Here, the broth is made with shiitake mushrooms instead of kombu. It is important to use whole, dried shiitake—fresh mushrooms do not give the same deep umami taste. You can find dried shiitake in Asian grocery stores.

2 SERVINGS
6 whole, dried shiitake mushrooms
2½ cups water
1 sweet potato
⅔ cup frozen shelled edamame (soybeans)
¼ cup white miso paste (instant miso powder also works in a pinch)
7 oz firm tofu

TO GARNISH
2 scallions

Brush the mushrooms carefully; do not rinse them. Put into a large airtight jar, pour in the measured water, and seal. Let soak in the refrigerator for at least 4 hours, preferably overnight, to extract all the flavor.

Peel the sweet potato, then cut into cubes. Remove the mushrooms from the soaking water and set aside. Add the mushroom soaking water and sweet potato cubes to a large saucepan. Bring to a boil, then reduce the heat and simmer for about 5 minutes, until the potatoes soften. Add the edamame (soybeans) 1 minute before the end of the cooking time.

Take a little of the hot broth and mix with the miso in a separate bowl. Pour the miso mixture into the soup in the pan and keep it warm but not boiling.

Cut the tofu into cubes. Add the tofu and reserved whole mushrooms to the miso soup so they warm through a little.

Coarsley chop the scallions. Ladle the soup into 2 bowls and garnish with the scallions.

Saikyo yaki—miso-glazed salmon

The first thing I do every time I'm back in Tokyo is hunt down saikyo yaki, a firm fish that has been marinated for a long time in sweet white miso (saikyo miso), mirin, and sake and then roasted. It becomes sweet, salty, and indescribably delicious. To sit under the glow of a red lantern with a piece of saikyo yaki clasped in chopsticks is happiness for me, and it is my constant partner in crime on my life's culinary journey for my skin. If you can't find saikyo miso, which is slightly sweet in taste, add some extra honey to the marinade.

4–5 SERVINGS
1 cup saikyo miso or white miso paste
½ cup mirin
¼ cup sake
1 tablespoon toasted sesame oil (optional)
1¾ pounds salmon (preferably
    sashimi-grade)

TO GARNISH
black sesame seeds
scallion

TO SERVE
pickled ginger (gari)
brown rice (genmai) (optional)
salad (optional)

Start 1 or 2 days before serving the food. Whisk together the miso, mirin, sake, and sesame oil, if using, then transfer about 3 tablespoons of the marinade to a separate bowl and reserve for the day you serve the dish. Put the salmon in a nonreactive dish (preferably one with a lid) and cover it completely with the remaining marinade so that the fish absorbs all the flavors.

Cover the dish with plastic wrap and seal with the lid (so that the smell won't escape) and put into the refrigerator.

On D-day, preheat the oven to 400°F. Gently wipe away and discard the excess marinade from the fish, because it can burn. Transfer the fish to a roasting pan lined with parchment paper and bake in the middle of the oven for 10 minutes, until just cooked through. Remove the fish from the oven and preheat the broiler. Brush the reserved marinade over the salmon and cook under the broiler until the surface is crisp and golden.

Sprinkle with sesame seeds and shredded scallion. Serve with pickled ginger and maybe a little brown rice or salad.

TIP!
It's important the salmon used here is top quality. I love salmon. Don't skimp on quality. If you really want to pump up the marinade, add a little grated ginger, crushed garlic, or honey.

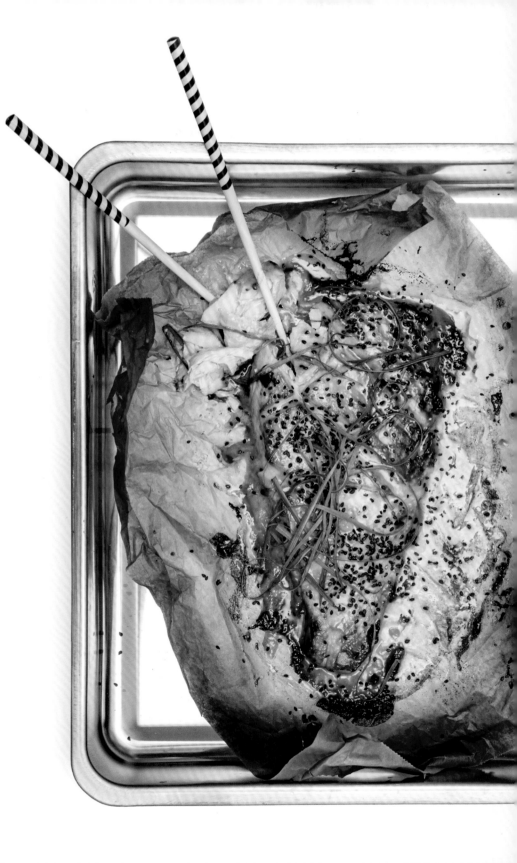

Steamed edamame (soybeans)

If you come to dinner at my home, edamame (soybeans) are always served with predinner drinks. Ice-cold umeshu (plum wine) with club soda is my dream companion on a hot summer's evening, but well-chilled bubbles and white wine are, of course, just as good. But for heaven's sake, buy whole edamame, where the beans remain in their cozy pods. A friend who I once asked to bring edamame to have with drinks brought a package of shelled edamame. Chewing the beans out of the salted pods is half the fun. If you can get fresh edamame in an Asian grocery store, you can consider yourself lucky.

4 SERVINGS

**4 cups frozen edamame (soybeans) in their pods
generous pinch of good-quality sea salt flakes or
    a pinch of togarashi (a Japanese chili blend)**

Cook the beans according to the package directions, but be careful to avoid overcooking them, because edamame should be served al dente. Refresh in ice-cold water, then drain thoroughly. Serve sprinkled with the salt or togarashi.

BEAUTY BONUS NO. 31

Edamame (soybeans) are not only one of the world's best snacks but they also slow down the breakdown of collagen. Prime wrinkle defense in a little pod!

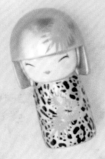

Salmon and avocado poke bowl

For the Japanese, a vacation in Hawaii is the equivalent of a vacation in the Canary Islands for us Swedes, and during Japan's Golden Week—the mandatory annual spring break, when all major companies shut down business to force the loyal workforce to go on vacation—our little family also took a trip over the Pacific. In Japan, we often ate chirashi (sushi on a bed of rice), but during the weeks in Maui and Honolulu, we came across the Hawaiian variant called "poke." I have still never eaten poke in Japan, but during my last trip, I discovered the phenomenon of millefeuille ("thousand-layer") sushi, where fish, rice, and avocado are layered in a glass jar. You heard it here first!

2 SERVINGS
1 cup short-grain brown rice
7 oz sashimi-grade salmon
1–2 scallions
2 avocados

MARINADE
¼ cup tamari or Japanese soy sauce
2 teaspoons rice vinegar
1 tablespoon toasted sesame oil

TOPPING
pickled ginger (gari)
unhulled white or black sesame seeds
pea shoot

Cook the rice according to the package directions. Whisk together all the marinade ingredients in a bowl.

Cut the fish into cubes, about ½ × ½ inch, and thinly slice the scallions. Put into a nonreactive bowl and pour over the marinade. Stir carefully so all the salmon pieces are coated. Marinate for 5 minutes.

Cut the avocados into cubes. Drain the rice, then put into 2 bowls. Top with the salmon, avocado, and pickled ginger. Sprinkle with sesame seeds and garnish with a pea shoot.

TIP!
Enhance the poke bowl with shredded winter radish, fermented carrots, edamame (soybeans), shredded nori, furikake, or sesame-marinated wakame seaweed.

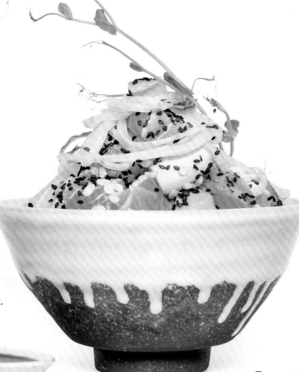

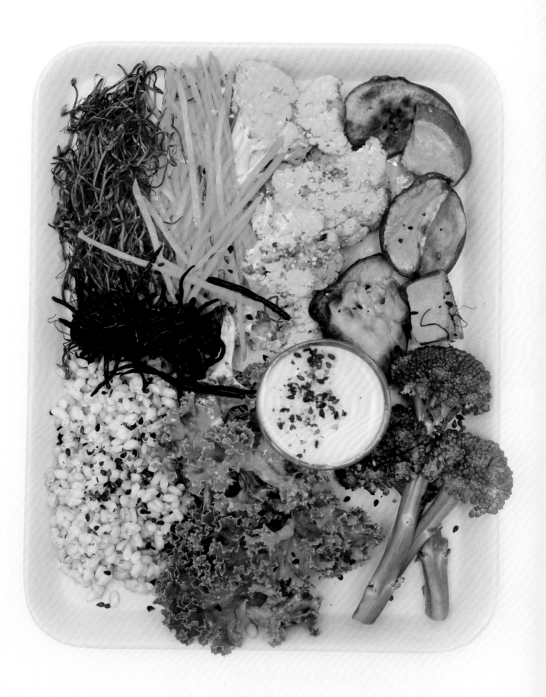

Macro bowls—Japanese bowl food

While low-carb high-fat diets and carbohydrate anxiety raged across Sweden, I sat on the other side of the planet, eating rice daily—and I had never felt better (my skin agrees). Genmai (short-grain brown rice) is the basis of the macrobiotic food philosophy. When I moved to Tokyo in 2007, there were rows of macrobiotic cafés in exclusive neighborhoods, and takeout boxes containing seaweed salad, brown onigiri rice balls, or soba noodles were standard at every *conbini* (convenience store).

Even outside Japan, the macrobiotic trend sprang up. Madonna became so smitten by it that she employed a Japanese cook, Mayumi Nishimura, who for seven years filled the pop queen with brown rice and whole grains, vegetables, seaweed, miso, fermented goodies, tofu, and occasionally some fish. And because, according to macrobiotic philosophy, it takes seven years for all the cells to be replaced, Mayumi Nishimura has effectively rebuilt Madonna's body.

Hard-core supporters of macrobiotic eating calculate their daily food intake with mathematical precision:

Whole grains and rice	40–60 percent
Vegetables	20–30 percent
Beans, tofu, and other bean products	5–10 percent
Algae (such as seaweed)	2 percent

But I don't really agree with this. When I interviewed Mayumi Nishimura, she told me about "petit macro"—picking parts of the macrobiotic philosophy to follow in everyday life without forbidding anything. I like that! We are beauty foodies, not ascetics. And yes, even Madonna eats brownies.

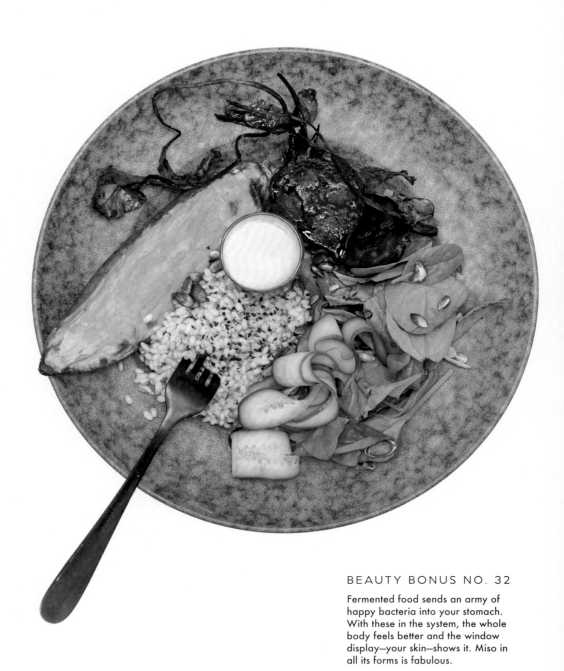

BEAUTY BONUS NO. 32

Fermented food sends an army of
happy bacteria into your stomach.
With these in the system, the whole
body feels better and the window
display—your skin—shows it. Miso in
all its forms is fabulous.

Macro bowl with roasted beet, sweet potato, and sweet-and-sour orange and miso dressing

The combination of the sweetness in the roasted beet and sweet potato and the salt in the pumpkin seeds is crazy good. The dressing with miso and orange really makes it special.

2 SERVINGS

1¼ cups short-grain brown rice
   or 1½ cups quinoa
1 large or 2 small sweet potatoes
2 raw red beets
2 teaspoons coconut oil
⅓ cup pumpkin seeds
½ cucumber
2 cups baby spinach
sea salt flakes

SWEET-AND-SOUR ORANGE
AND MISO DRESSING
3 tablespoons white miso paste
3 tablespoons tahini
finely grated zest of 1 orange
3 tablespoons orange juice
1 tablespoon olive oil
2 teaspoons honey or maple syrup
2 teaspoons tamari soy sauce
½–1 tablespoon grated fresh ginger
   (press out the juice)

TOPPING
toasted pumpkin seeds
gomashio (see page 103)

Preheat the oven to 400°F. Cook the rice or quinoa according to the package directions. Mix together all ingredients for the dressing, adding a little water if it is too thick, then set aside.

Meanwhile, wash and scrub the sweet potatoes and beets, then cut them in half. Gently melt the coconut oil in a small saucepan. Coat the root vegetables in the melted oil and sprinkle with salt. Transfer to a roasting pan lined with a sheet of parchment paper and bake in the middle of the oven for at least 30 minutes (turning them over halfway through the cooking time, if you want), or until the vegetables are golden on the outside and tender all the way through.

Toast the pumpkin seeds with a little salt in a dry skillet over medium heat until golden. Transfer to a plate and let cool. Cut the cucumber into thin ribbons with a potato peeler.

Arrange the baby spinach, drained rice, roasted root vegetables, and cucumber in a bowl. Serve with the dressing and sprinkle over a little toasted pumpkin seeds and gomashio.

Summer macro plate à la Brown Rice Café

On a backstreet off Tokyo's version of Rodeo Drive, Omotesando, is one of my favorite little oases on the earth—Brown Rice Café. It follows the macrobiotic food philosophy and every day a new *seto*, the Japanese equivalent of the daily special, is served with side dishes. One summer's day, when a humid Tokyo heat was hanging over the city, a simple but oh so delicious salad with soba noodles and summer vegetables was served. This is my variation, but you can build it with whatever vegetables you happen to have at home. I've left out the quantities so you can customize it according to what you have or how many will be eating.

2 SERVINGS
soba noodles
carrots
red cabbage
red bell pepper and yellow bell pepper
cucumber
firm tofu, preferably pressed (see page 86)
pea shoots
white sesame seeds

DIPPING SAUCE
2 tablespoons shoyu
2 tablespoons mirin
1 tablespoon rice vinegar
½ cup dashi (see page 87) or water
1 teaspoon sesame oil

First make the sauce. Heat the shoyu, mirin, rice vinegar, and dashi or water in a medium saucepan. It should not boil. Remove from the heat and let cool, then whisk in the sesame oil.

Cook the noodles according to the package directions, then drain and let cool before serving. Peel the carrots. Shred the red cabbage and cut the carrots, bell peppers, and cucumber into long matchsticks. Cut the tofu into cubes. Arrange the noodles and vegetables in a large bowl. Sprinkle over sesame seeds and serve with the sauce.

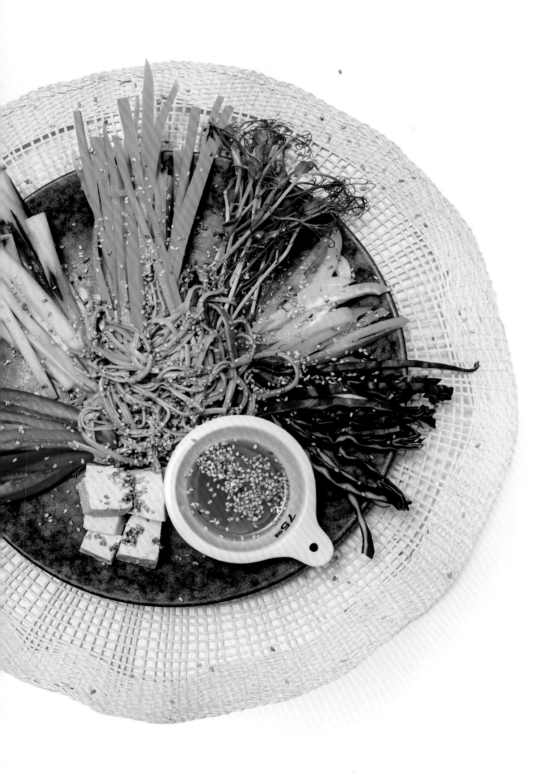

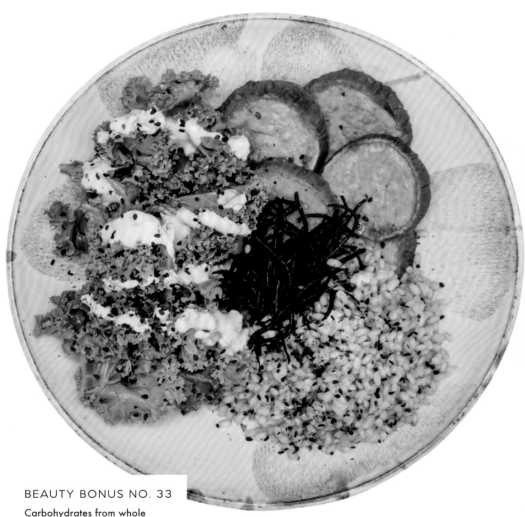

BEAUTY BONUS NO. 33

Carbohydrates from whole grains won't hurt you. Just the opposite—brown rice and other grains are rocket fuel for beauty. And no, they won't make you fat.

Macro bowl with roasted sweet potato, lemony sesame kale, arame seaweed, and tahini dressing

A plate with several sections is fun to explore, especially when each section, or station, if you will, holds a whole world of beauty. A brown rice station, vegetable station, seaweed station, dressing station, and a station of something hearty all lead to the final stop: GLOW. To bring the dish to complete perfection, top it with gomashio—a crazy-good Japanese beauty topping of black sesame seeds and sea salt flakes. Grind three portions of black sesame seeds to one portion of salt into a coarse powder.

2 SERVINGS
¾ oz dried arame seaweed
1 large or 2 small sweet potatoes
½ tablespoon coconut oil
1¼ cups short-grain brown rice
a few generous handfuls of kale
juice of 1 lemon
½ tablespoon sesame oil
black sesame seeds or gomashio
sea salt flakes

MISO AND TAHINI DRESSING WITH LEMON
3 tablespoons tahini
1 tablespoon white miso paste
2 tablespoons water, warmed but not boiling
juice of 1 lemon
1 tablespoon grated fresh ginger
2 teaspoons maple syrup (optional)

Soak the arame according to the package directions, then drain. Preheat the oven to 400°F. Scrub the sweet potato, then cut into rounds and put onto a large baking sheet lined with parchment paper.

Gently melt the coconut oil in a small saucepan, then coat the sweet potato rounds in the melted oil and sprinkle with salt. Roast in the middle of the oven for about 30 minutes, until the pieces are golden and tender.

Meanwhile, cook the rice according to the package directions. Tear the kale into large pieces and put into a large bowl. Pour over the lemon juice and sesame oil and massage the cabbage until it softens.

Mix together all the dressing ingredients until smooth, adding a little more water if the dressing is too thick.

Arrange the kale, drained rice, and sweet potatoes in a large bowl. Add the well-drained arame. Drizzle with the dressing and sprinkle over black sesame seeds or gomashio.

Friday face food

Beauty-proofed cocktails and snacks

Snacks and cocktails are a part of life, and should, of course, be part of a beauty routine. Because we are beauty foodies and not ascetics, we don't stay at home with green juice when the weekend finally arrives. It's possible to have a beauty-proofed Friday celebration and swig an adult drink when the mood strikes. Put on your eyelashes and a party hat, because here we go!

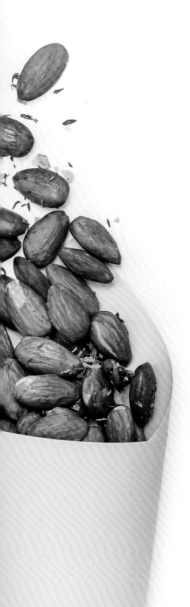

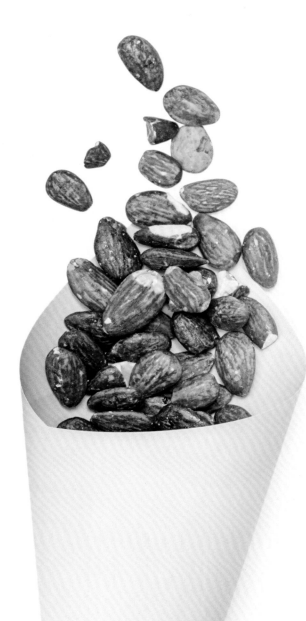

THYME-ROASTED ALMONDS
RECIPE ON PAGE 111

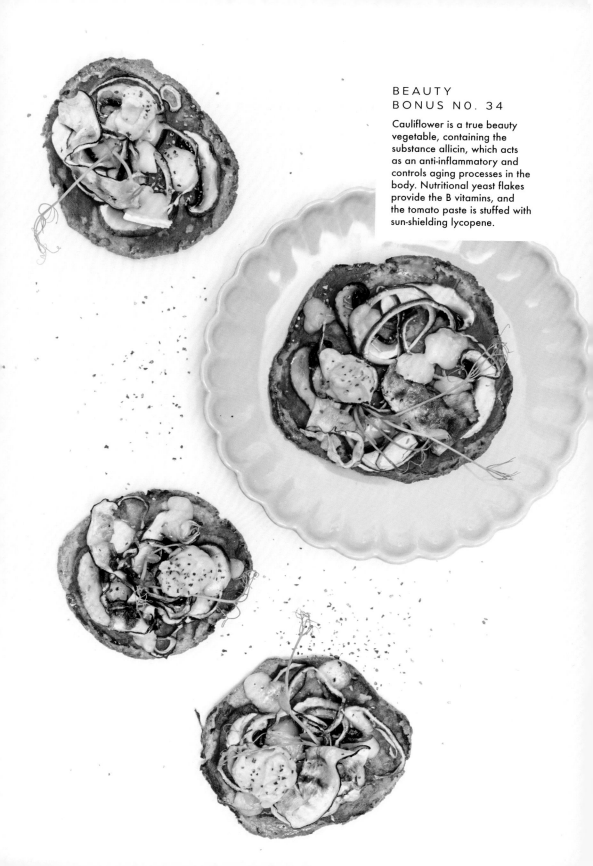

Cauliflower mini-pizzas with avocado cream

I'll be honest. This pizza is really best for a day when you have the time and energy to spend a little longer in the kitchen, and for me, that day is rarely Friday. Dealing with cauliflower rice is . . . well, crumbly. But sometimes it happens. We turn up the party music in our little kitchen and fill our glasses with rich red wine. And when you sit with a crisp, 100 percent beauty-proofed pizza in your palm, it's worth the work. In many cauliflower recipes, grated cheese is used in the dough, but I go with nutritional yeast flakes to get that cheesy flavor and a hearty dose of the hair-loving B vitamins.

5 SMALL PIZZAS

PIZZA CRUST DOUGH
1 small or ¾ large cauliflower
(makes about 4 cups cauliflower rice)
1 egg
¾ cup plus 2 tablespoons almond flour
1¼ cups buckwheat flour
¾ cup nutritional yeast flakes
1 teaspoon dried oregano
1 teaspoon dried thyme
1 teaspoon dried rosemary
1 teaspoon salt

AVOCADO CREAM
1 large ripe avocado
2 garlic cloves
2 tablespoons lemon juice
1 teaspoon chili flakes
salt

TOPPING
15 cremini mushrooms
1 zucchini
1 red onion
¼ cup tomato paste

OPTIONAL PIZZA TOPPINGS
arugula
pea shoots
sliced ripe black olives
hemp seeds

Preheat the oven to 400°F. Cut the cauliflower florets into small pieces and process in a food processor to a ricelike consistency. Steam the cauliflower rice for 7 minutes—this will help you to squeeze out more liquid. Let the cauliflower cool, then transfer it onto dry paper towels (or into a nut milk bag, if you have one) and squeeze out all the liquid. It takes about 2 minutes before it is dry enough. Don't cheat and skip this step!

Beat the egg. Mix the almond flour, buckwheat flour, nutritional yeast flakes, oregano, thyme, rosemary, and salt into a mound. Add the cauliflower and beaten egg. Mix together, then knead to a dough. Divide into 5 equal balls, then press them into round pizza crusts, the thinner the better (some olive oil on the hands can make this process easier). Place on a baking sheet lined with parchment paper. Bake in the middle of the oven for about 20 minutes.

Mash the avocado, crushed garlic, and lemon juice to a completely smooth, fluffy cream. Stir in the chili flakes and season with salt. Put in the refrigerator.

Slice the mushrooms thinly. Using a potato peeler, slice the zucchini into ribbons. Peel the onion, then slice into thin rings. Remove the pizza crusts from the oven. Spread with the tomato paste, then top with the mushrooms, zucchini ribbons, and onion. Return to the oven and cook for another 15 minutes, until the onion and mushrooms are roasted. Personally, I like crispy, almost burned edges, so sometimes I let my pizzas bake a little longer.

Remove the pizzas from the oven. Let cool, then add a spoonful of the avocado cream. Serve topped with your choice of arugula, pea shoots, olives, and/ or hemp seeds.

Sour cream 'n' onion kale chips

For many years, I traveled to London or New York with half-empty suitcases in order to ship home (horribly expensive) bags of kale chips from Whole Foods. Then I found some retailers in Stockholm, and the decade's most expensive habit gained momentum. After some anxiety-producing bank statements, I decided to become a kale chips master. And I think I've managed it well! As an onion lover, I add a lot of onion granules. Enjoy the chips with ice-cold white wine.

3–4 SERVINGS

1½ cups cashew nuts
10½ oz kale (preferably on the stem)
3 tablespoons nutritional yeast flakes
2 tablespoons water
2 tablespoons onion powder or granules
1 tablespoon apple cider vinegar
1 tablespoon olive or canola oil
juice of 1 lemon
1 teaspoon garlic powder (optional)
2 teaspoons sea salt flakes, plus extra
  for sprinking

Soak the cashew nuts in water for at least 30 minutes. Preheat the oven to 300°F. Rinse the kale, then pat dry with paper towels—this is really crucial, because the smallest droplet of water makes for boring soggy chips. Gently tear the leaves from the stem. The perfect chip is about 2 × 2 inches. Put into a large bowl.

Drain the cashew nuts, then rinse thoroughly. Blend the nuts with the other ingredients to a cream in a high-speed blender, adding extra water if the mixture is too thick. Pour the cream over the kale, then massage it in for at least 1 minute, until all the leaves are coated.

Spread the kale on baking sheets lined with parchment paper, leaving a small amount of space between the leaves. You can have 2 sheets inside the oven at the same time. Bake the chips for 25–35 minutes, until the cashew cream is crunchily golden and the chips are crisp but not burned. Remove the sheets after about 15 minutes and turn the chips so that they bake evenly for the remaining time. Remove from the oven, sprinkle with some extra salt, and let cool before serving.

TIP!
Rinse the kale the day before and dry the leaves on paper towels in the refrigerator overnight.

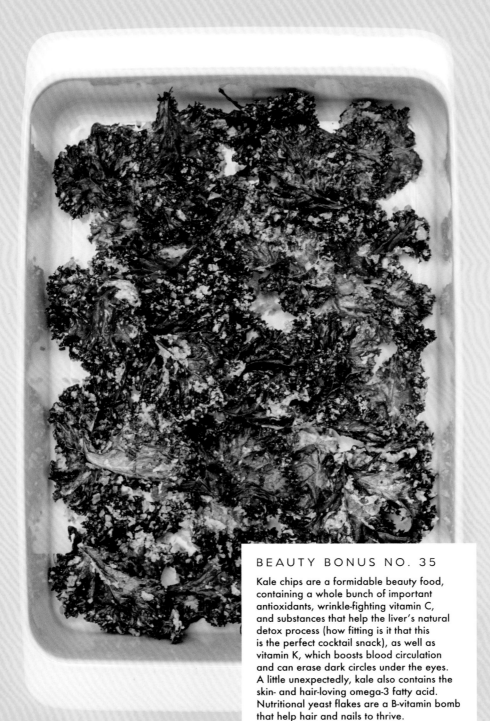

BEAUTY BONUS NO. 35

Kale chips are a formidable beauty food, containing a whole bunch of important antioxidants, wrinkle-fighting vitamin C, and substances that help the liver's natural detox process (how fitting is it that this is the perfect cocktail snack), as well as vitamin K, which boosts blood circulation and can erase dark circles under the eyes. A little unexpectedly, kale also contains the skin- and hair-loving omega-3 fatty acid. Nutritional yeast flakes are a B-vitamin bomb that help hair and nails to thrive.

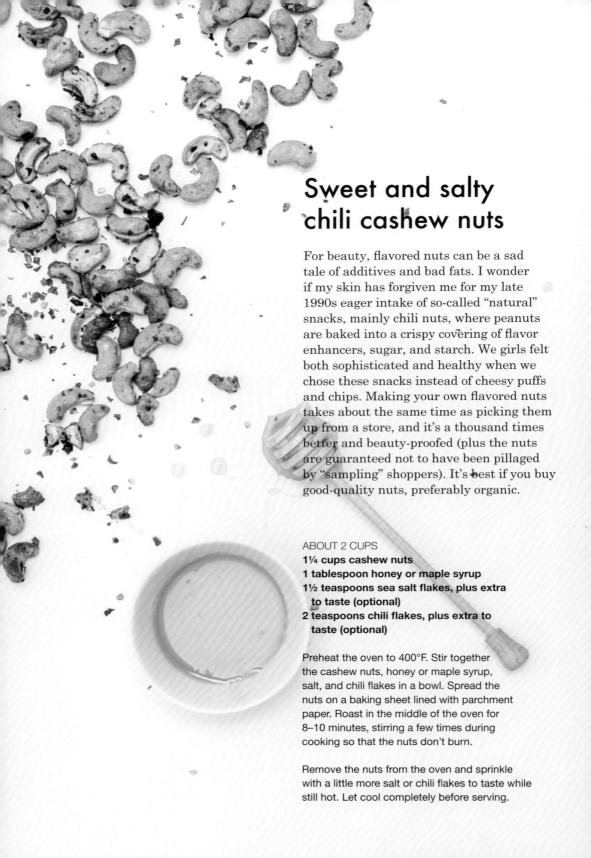

Sweet and salty chili cashew nuts

For beauty, flavored nuts can be a sad tale of additives and bad fats. I wonder if my skin has forgiven me for my late 1990s eager intake of so-called "natural" snacks, mainly chili nuts, where peanuts are baked into a crispy covering of flavor enhancers, sugar, and starch. We girls felt both sophisticated and healthy when we chose these snacks instead of cheesy puffs and chips. Making your own flavored nuts takes about the same time as picking them up from a store, and it's a thousand times better and beauty-proofed (plus the nuts are guaranteed not to have been pillaged by "sampling" shoppers). It's best if you buy good-quality nuts, preferably organic.

ABOUT 2 CUPS
1¼ cups cashew nuts
1 tablespoon honey or maple syrup
1½ teaspoons sea salt flakes, plus extra to taste (optional)
2 teaspoons chili flakes, plus extra to taste (optional)

Preheat the oven to 400°F. Stir together the cashew nuts, honey or maple syrup, salt, and chili flakes in a bowl. Spread the nuts on a baking sheet lined with parchment paper. Roast in the middle of the oven for 8–10 minutes, stirring a few times during cooking so that the nuts don't burn.

Remove the nuts from the oven and sprinkle with a little more salt or chili flakes to taste while still hot. Let cool completely before serving.

Thyme-roasted almonds

If you feel up to it, you can blanch and peel the almonds, but I keep the skins on. Replace the thyme with dried rosemary for variety. If you want some bite, a little smoked paprika powder is good in the mix. As I'm writing this, it's New Year's Eve, and what do you think is in the oven and spreading the most wonderful aroma right now? I see it as my duty that all guests' skin starts the New Year in the best possible way.

ABOUT 2 CUPS
1 cup whole almonds
½ tablespoon olive oil
1 tablespoon dried thyme
1½ teaspoons sea salt flakes

Preheat the oven to 350°F. Mix together the almonds, olive oil, thyme, and salt. Spread the nuts on a baking sheet lined with parchment paper. Roast them in the oven on a high shelf for 12–15 minutes, until they are golden. Stir around during this time and keep an eye on them to make sure they don't burn. Let cool before serving.

BEAUTY BONUS NO. 36

Almonds boast one of nature's highest contents of vitamin E, which helps prevent the effects of beauty-sabotaging free radicals.

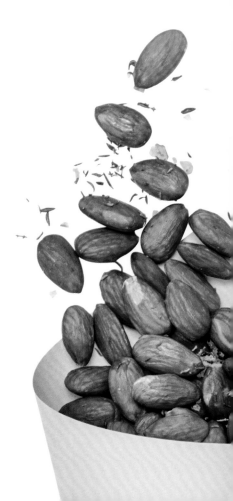

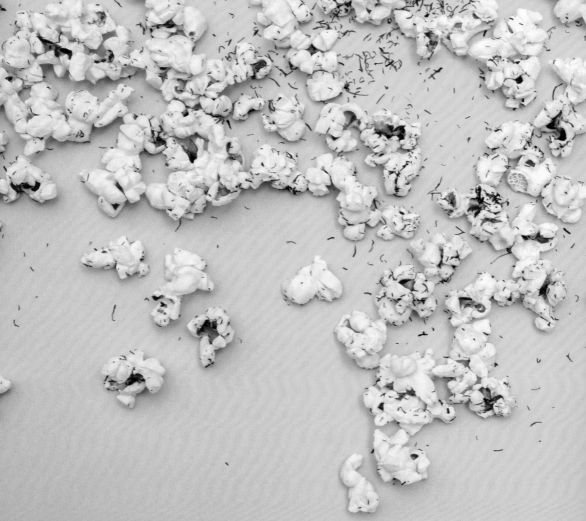

Dill popcorn

It isn't a party without popcorn!
Pop the kernels in coconut oil and
you have a super snack to chill
with and a snow white conscience.
My mother-in-law gave me a jar
of dried dill sprouts, made by the
brand Herbaria, and since then,
I constantly have a craving for dill.
In general, the store-bought dried
herb can be a little boring, and you
might not find dried dill sprouts,
so use chopped fresh dill instead.

1 LARGE BOWL
1½–2 tablespoons coconut oil
½ cup popping corn
a generous pinch of salt or herb salt
1–2 tablespoons chopped fresh dill

Melt the coconut oil in a saucepan over the
highest heat until the melted oil completely
covers the bottom of the pan. Add some of the
corn kernels and cover the pan with the lid. When
it starts to pop, add the remaining corn kernels in
a thin layer in the bottom of the pan. Replace the
lid and reduce the heat slightly when the popping
is in full swing. When you can count to five
between the pops, remove the pan from the heat.
Remove the lid when the popping completely
stops. Sprinkle with the salt and dill, replace the
lid, shake to coat all the popcorn, then serve.

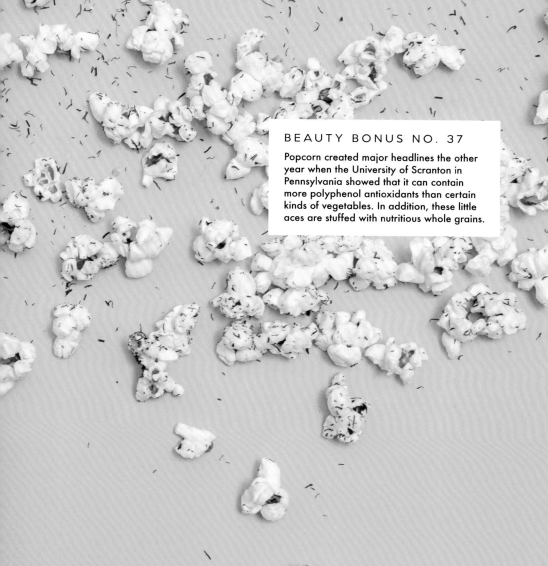

BEAUTY BONUS NO. 37

Popcorn created major headlines the other year when the University of Scranton in Pennsylvania showed that it can contain more polyphenol antioxidants than certain kinds of vegetables. In addition, these little aces are stuffed with nutritious whole grains.

BEAUTY
BONUS NO. 38

Kombucha is a fermented tea drink
with beauty-promoting antioxidants,
enzymes, and good bacteria that
make the stomach happy. Buy
raw kombucha that has not been
pasteurized, so you can be sure
that the nutrients are intact.

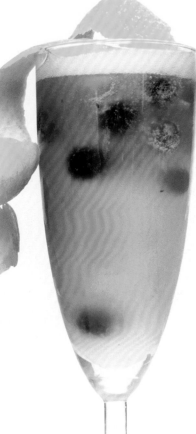

Ginger kombucha fizzle

The fermented tea beverage kombucha
isn't just incredibly nutritious. It also
has a festive fizz effect when drinking
it. And fizzle = giggle, which is always
good. Look for kombucha flavored with
ginger in combination with lemon or
apple. Unbelievably good.

1 GLASS
a few frozen blueberries
2 tablespoons lemon juice
1 teaspoon agave syrup
2 tablespoons plus 2 teaspoons gin
   (1½ oz)
¾ cup ice-cold kombucha flavored with
   apple and ginger or lemon and ginger
ice cube (optional)

Put the blueberries into the bottom of a
champagne glass. Pour in the lemon juice,
agave syrup, and gin. Top off with the
kombucha. Add an ice cube, if liked, and
decorate with a lemon twist.

Coconut glowjito

Here, I've upgraded a traditional mojito to a beauty-proofed glowjito. Lime, mint, and coconut water are a supertrio, not only because the flavors marry together like a dream, but also because together they fill the body with vitamin C and moisturizing electrolytes. You can often find large bunches of fresh mint at Asian food stores, if not at your local grocery store.

1 GLASS OR JAR
2 limes
a generous handful of mint—don't
  be stingy
½ tablespoon agave syrup
3 tablespoons plus 2 teaspoons
  white rum (1½ oz)
½ cup coconut water
crushed ice
½ club soda

Squeeze the juice from 1 of the limes into a large and stable glass or cocktail jar. Thoroughly wash the other lime, cut it into 4–6 wedges, and put into the glass. Tear in the mint leaves and drizzle in the agave syrup. Muddle the lime and mint together with a pestle, wooden spoon, or special cocktail muddler until they are well crushed. Pour in the rum, coconut water, and ice, then stir. Top off with the club soda.

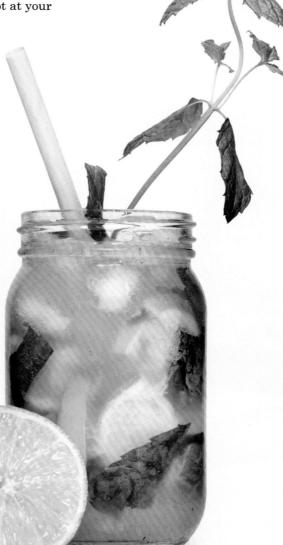

Orlando's Jamaican pineapple chow

Lina, the photographer who took the pictures for this book, for some years now has been running a Caribbean summer bar, Orlando's Jamaican, on Gotland island, Sweden. Their pineapple chow, a kind of superchunky pineapple salsa, is really good and a delight, not least for us beauty hunters. Adjust the chili to taste.

2–3 SERVINGS
1 pineapple
a generous handful of cilantro, plus
   extra leaves to decorate
½ red chili, plus extra to decorate
juice of 2 limes
sea salt flakes

Peel the pineapple and slice into bite-size cubes. Finely chop the cilantro and chili, then mix together with the lime juice. Put the pineapple into a bowl and pour over the marinade. Sprinkle with salt and top with extra cilantro leaves and chili slices.

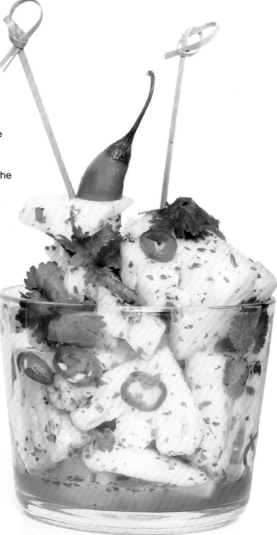

Frozen strawberry daiquiri

Cocktail hour does not have to spoil the beauty celebration. Bring out your fancy lipstick and party high heels, and treat your skin to a well-deserved rest at the beauty bar. After all, it's Friday! This sour strawberry dream is stuffed with vitamin C that positively invites the collagen to dance.

1 GLASS
2 tablespoons plus 2 teaspoons
  light rum (1½ oz)
8 frozen strawberries, partly
  defrosted, plus extra if required
¼ cup coconut water, plus extra if required
juice of 1 lime
1 teaspoon agave syrup
3–4 ice cubes

TO DECORATE
fresh strawberries

Blend the rum, slightly defrosted strawberries, coconut water, lime juice, agave syrup, and ice in a high-speed blender until well combined. Add extra strawberries for a sorbetlike consistency, or more coconut water if the blades have trouble spinning. Pour into a cocktail glass and decorate with some whole fresh strawberries.

Beauty brunch

Waffles, pancakes, and other Sunday comfort foods

After Friday face food, of course, it's time for
a blow-out beauty brunch with pancakes, waffles,
and rolls on the menu. Sunday blues don't have
a chance against that. It's also guaranteed to be
Instagram friendly.

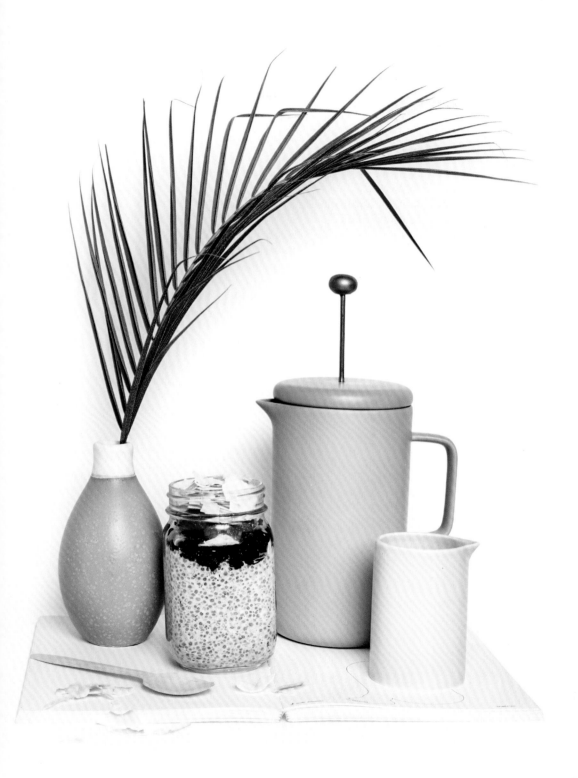

Banana pancakes with chia preserves

Everyone loves pancakes, including my little family. Without a doubt, pancakes are the dish served most often at home. They are loved by the discerning child, the beauty food mother, and the protein-eating, lycra-wearing athlete father, who deserves the credit for bringing banana pancakes into our home when his midlife crisis introduced him to the world of muscles and marathons. A tip from the athletes: Take advantage of the time when the cakes are cooking to do some kettlebell swings. Several times I've been met by the sight of my bare-chested husband bumping against the stove (the sideboard hides the kettlebell from view, so all I see is a half-naked man grinding away—a sight I could do without). I prefer to skip all the bumping and grinding, but I'm childishly fond of building a pancake stack with preserves, coconut cream, chocolate sauce, and fresh berries.

12 PANCAKES
2 large ripe bananas
6 eggs
⅔ cup almond flour
¼ cup plant-based milk
pinch of vanilla powder
pinch of ground cinnamon
coconut oil, for frying

RAW CHOCOLATE SAUCE (OPTIONAL)
½ cup coconut oil at room temperature
  (if it becomes too runny, put into the
  refrigerator for a few minutes)
¼ cup yacon syrup
3 tablespoons raw cacao
2 teaspoons vanilla powder

TO SERVE
Coconut Whipped Cream (see recipe
  on page 125)
Chia Preserves (see recipes on page 122)
fresh berries
fresh fruit
toasted coconut chips

Peel the bananas and slice them into small rounds. Using a handheld blender, blend the bananas with the eggs, almond flour, milk, vanilla, and cinnamon until the batter is airy. Let stand for about 10 minutes.

To make the chocolate sauce, stir together all the ingredients until smooth. Set aside.

Heat the coconut oil in a small skillet over medium heat, add a little of the batter, and cook until the pancake is golden brown on both sides (you'll be able to flip it once it's no longer runny). Repeat to make 12 pancakes. Serve with your choice of the following: chocolate sauce, Coconut Whipped Cream, Chia Preserves, plenty of berries and other fruit, and toasted coconut chips.

BEAUTY BONUS NO. 39

Eggs are rocket fuel for beauty, packed with protein, vitamin B₁₂, and biotin, which benefits skin, hair, and nails. Banana is rich in potassium, which is a superweapon against water retention, including bags under the eyes. Berries, overflowing with antioxidants, are like small capsules of the world's best antiaging serum that protects the skin cells.

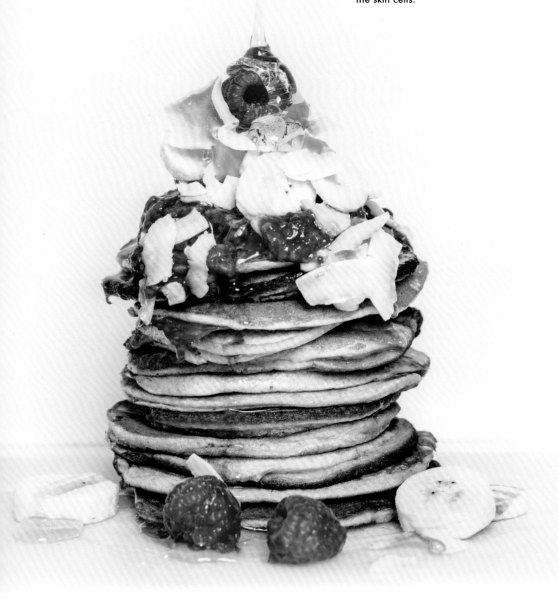

Three types of beautifying chia preserves

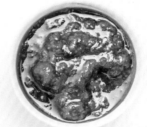

RASPBERRY CHIA PRESERVES
1 cup frozen raspberries
3 tablespoons chia seeds
1 tablespoon coconut nectar
1 teaspoon vanilla powder

BLUEBERRY CHIA PRESERVES
1½ cups frozen blueberries
3 tablespoons chia seeds
1 tablespoon coconut nectar
1 teaspoon vanilla powder
1 teaspoon ground cinnamon or
    ground cardamom (optional)

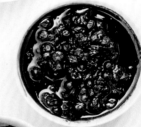

CHERRY CHIA PRESERVES
1½ cups frozen cherries
3 tablespoons chia seeds
1 tablespoons coconut nectar
1 teaspoon vanilla powder

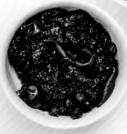

Defrost or warm the berries or cherries until they just start to soften, then mash with a fork until they release their juices.

Stir in the chia seeds, coconut nectar, vanilla powder and cinnamon or cardamom, if liked. Refrigerate for at least 15 minutes.

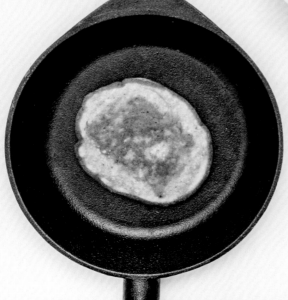

Overnight oats with chia, blueberries, and vanilla

A hybrid between overnight oats and chia pudding that's prepared the night before. Also perfect as a weekday breakfast.

4 SERVINGS
2 cups plant-based milk, plus extra to serve
1 cup fresh or defrosted blueberries
½ teaspoon vanilla powder
1 tablespoon yacon syrup or coconut nectar
3 cups oats
3 tablespoons chia seeds

TO SERVE
Chia Preserves (see opposite, optional)
fresh berries
toasted coconut chips

Using a handheld blender, blend the milk, blueberries, vanilla, and yacon syrup or coconut nectar until smooth. Stir in the oats and chia seeds. Pour into 2 airtight containers and let soak in the refrigerator overnight. Stir before serving and add more milk as needed. Serve with Chia Preserves (if you like), berries, and coconut chips.

BEAUTY BONUS NO. 40

A handful of oats a day will give your hair incredible body. In our stressful age, hair loss and/or premature hair loss is common. The hair is, after all, the body's last priority when it comes to nourishment, and if we're stressed or sick, nutrition is distributed to more needy organs (I know, the body can be a bitch). Oats contain a fantastic supercocktail of the B vitamins and zinc, as well as fiber, which keeps blood sugar under control.

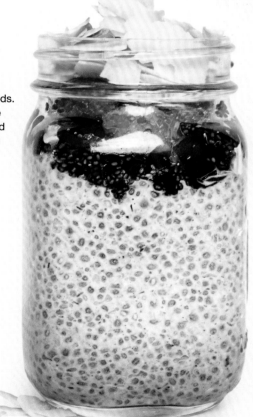

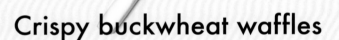

Crispy buckwheat waffles

Perfectly crispy, a touch sweet, and filled with beauty minerals from buckwheat flour. A brunch table VIP.

5 WAFFLES
2 cups buckwheat flour
1 teaspoon baking powder
1 teaspoon vanilla powder
1 teaspoon salt
1 cup plant-based milk
2 tablespoons yacon syrup or maple syrup
1 egg
1 teaspoon apple cider vinegar
3 tablespoons coconut oil

TO SERVE
fresh fruit
Chia Preserves (see recipes on page 122)
Coconut Whipped Cream (see opposite)

Preheat the waffle iron so that it has time to become really hot.

In a bowl, mix together the buckwheat, baking powder, vanilla powder, salt, milk, syrup, egg, and apple cider vinegar. Gently melt the coconut oil in a saucepan until it becomes just liquid, then stir into the batter. Mix thoroughly so that you don't get clumps (you can sift the buckwheat flour first if you're really ambitious). Cook the waffles in the waffle iron until golden.

Serve with fruit and Coconut Whipped Cream, or Chia Preserves.

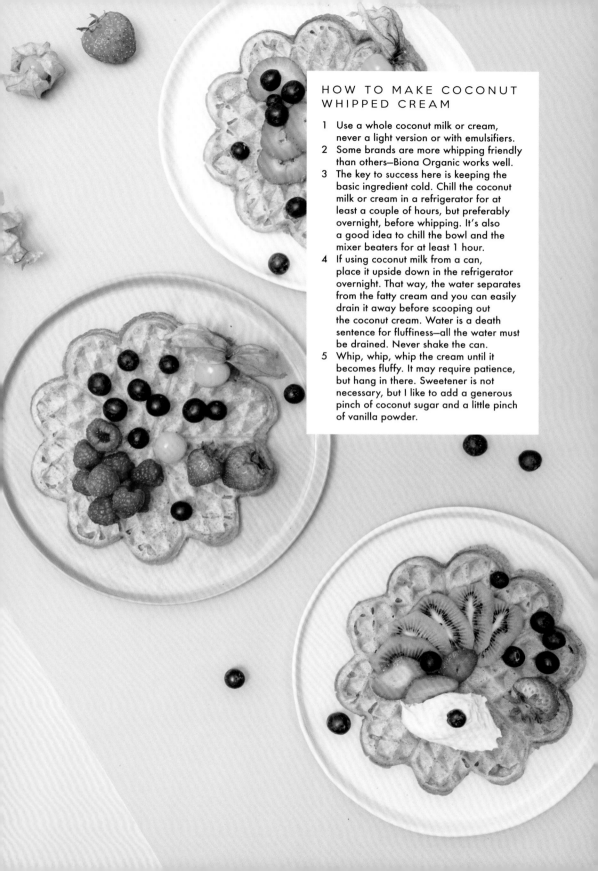

HOW TO MAKE COCONUT WHIPPED CREAM

1 Use a whole coconut milk or cream, never a light version or with emulsifiers.
2 Some brands are more whipping friendly than others—Biona Organic works well.
3 The key to success here is keeping the basic ingredient cold. Chill the coconut milk or cream in a refrigerator for at least a couple of hours, but preferably overnight, before whipping. It's also a good idea to chill the bowl and the mixer beaters for at least 1 hour.
4 If using coconut milk from a can, place it upside down in the refrigerator overnight. That way, the water separates from the fatty cream and you can easily drain it away before scooping out the coconut cream. Water is a death sentence for fluffiness—all the water must be drained. Never shake the can.
5 Whip, whip, whip the cream until it becomes fluffy. It may require patience, but hang in there. Sweetener is not necessary, but I like to add a generous pinch of coconut sugar and a little pinch of vanilla powder.

Cilla's magical spelt rolls

These brunch rolls were created by my colleague, Cilla. When she's not designing the *Lady's World* baking blog Homemade Stockholm, she's making sure that we editors never have our sweet cravings unresolved (she's a walking danger to the editors' skin, that Cilla). The rolls are made with whole-grain spelt flour, making them beauty-proofed. I love fennel seeds and I normally add some extra.

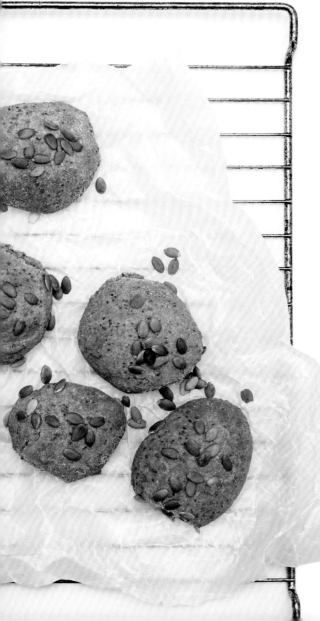

ABOUT 10 ROLLS
2 teaspoons dry active yeast
1⅔ cups cold water
1½ teaspoons salt
1 tablespoon honey
2 tablespoons coconut oil
1½ teaspoons fennel seeds
4½ cup whole-grain spelt flour, plus extra
 for dusting
¼ cup whole flaxseeds or chia seeds
2 tablespoons pumpkin seeds

Dissolve the yeast in the measured water, then mix into the salt, honey, coconut oil, finely crushed fennel seeds, and sifted spelt flour in a bowl. Stir with a plastic spatula, then add the flaxseeds or chia seeds. The dough does not need to be kneaded. Cover with plastic wrap and put into the refrigerator overnight.

Preheat the oven to 425°F. Pour ½ cup water into a baking pan and place at the bottom of the oven to create some steam, which gives a nice surface to the rolls.

Transfer the dough to a floured surface, divide it into 10 equal pieces, then shape into rolls and put onto a baking sheet lined with parchment paper. Sprinkle with the pumpkin seeds and a little flour. Let rise for 30 minutes, then bake in the middle of the oven for 20–25 minutes.

TOPPING SUGGESTIONS
avocado + chili flakes + sea salt flakes
smoked salmon + spinach leaves + squeezed
 lemon juice
mashed avocado + tomato + sea salt flakes
boiled egg + red bell pepper
Herbed Cashew Cream Cheese (see recipe
 opposite) + tomato

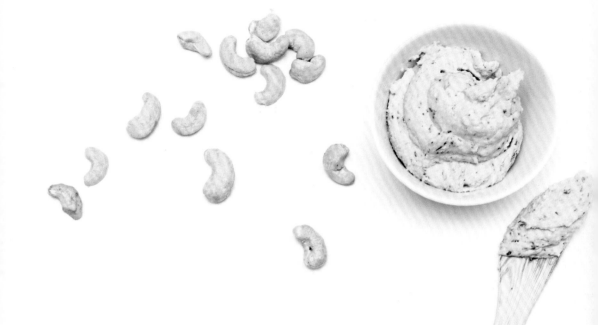

Herbed cashew cream cheese

ABOUT 1¼ CUPS
2 cups cashew nuts
juice of 1 lemon
1 tablespoon apple cider vinegar
2 tablespoons nutritional yeast flakes
1 teaspoon salt, preferably herb salt
2 cups finely chopped chives or dill, or
  a mix of both
¼ teaspoon black pepper

Soak the cashew nuts in water for at least
4 hours (but not too long, otherwise the nuts
become too wet). Drain welll.

Put the nuts, lemon juice, apple cider vinegar,
nutritional yeast flakes, and salt into a food
processor. Process to a perfectly smooth
"cheese"; this takes about 5 minutes. Stir in the
herbs and black pepper. Refrigerate and serve
cold. The cheese will keep for up to 5 days in an
airtight container in the refrigerator.

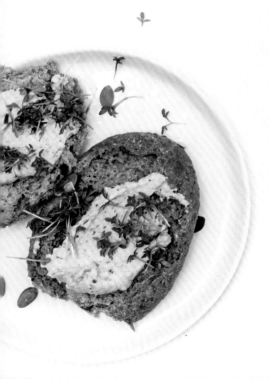

Nordic-style blueberry scones

The lemon gives an invigorating acidity and the coconut flour a wonderful sweetness. Make a double batch and freeze. Sometimes I toast them briefly to crisp the surface. If you want your scones to have the attractive cross on top (the trademark of Nordic-style scones) remove from the oven after about 10 minutes and gently score them, then return to the oven and continue to bake.

5 SCONES
½ cup frozen blueberries
1¼ cups almond flour
¾ cup plus 2 tablespoons coconut flour
3½ tablespoons coconut sugar
1 teaspoon baking powder
juice and finely grated zest of 1 lemon
1 tablespoon chia seeds
1 teaspoon ground cinnamon
1 teaspoon ground cardamom
¼ teaspoon salt
2 eggs
½ cup plant-based milk

Preheat the oven to 400°F. Defrost the blueberries and let drain so that the mixture isn't runny. Mix together the almond flour, coconut flour, coconut sugar, baking powder, lemon zest, chia seeds, cinnamon, cardamom, and salt in a large bowl.

Beat the eggs with the milk until fluffy, then stir in the lemon juice. Fold the egg mixture into the flour and spice mixture. Stir gently until everything is combined. Finally, stir in the blueberries with a spatula. Let stand for a minute.

Divide the dough into 5 equal pieces and shape into rounds. Flatten them well, making sure each scone is an even thickness. Place on a baking sheet lined with parchment paper and bake in the middle of the oven for 25–30 minutes, until golden and crispy at the edges.

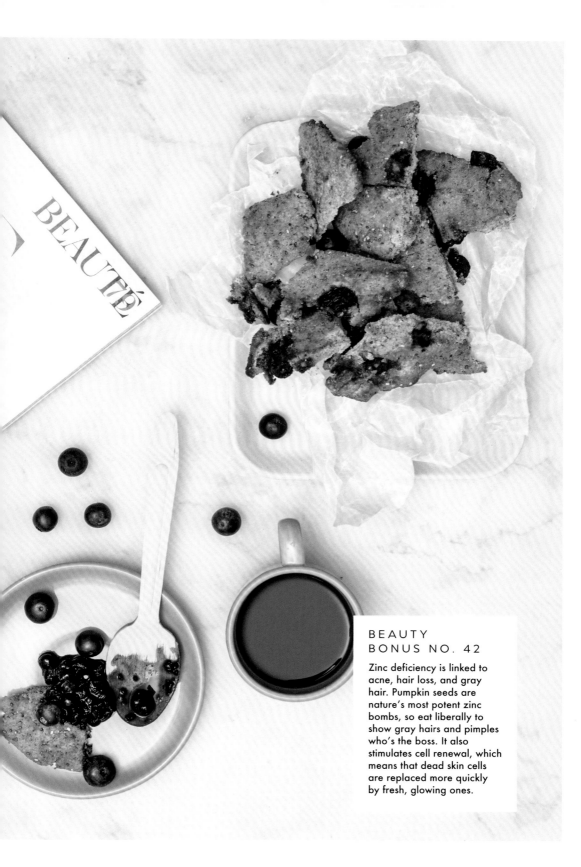

BEAUTY
BONUS NO. 42

Zinc deficiency is linked to acne, hair loss, and gray hair. Pumpkin seeds are nature's most potent zinc bombs, so eat liberally to show gray hairs and pimples who's the boss. It also stimulates cell renewal, which means that dead skin cells are replaced more quickly by fresh, glowing ones.

Sweet things

Desserts, cakes, and ice cream

Lipstick on the teeth and chocolate in the corners of the mouth are my trademark. Without these two companions, my teeth would be more white but my life would be gray. Nothing comforts my tattered soul, or relieves everything from Sunday blues to PMS-related crying sessions, like something creamy, chewy, and chocolaty (licking the bowl is well-documented crisis management). Chocolate is the best medicine for almost everything. To eat chocolate is to celebrate life. Ice cream, as well. Life is too short not to indulge a little. Treat yourself—a lot and often! And don't worry about whether you should or not; think of it as a human right. Every chew in this chapter is a declaration of love to you all. And an indispensable tip to all beauty foodie bakers—if the coconut oil is too hard, soften it up a little with a hair dryer.

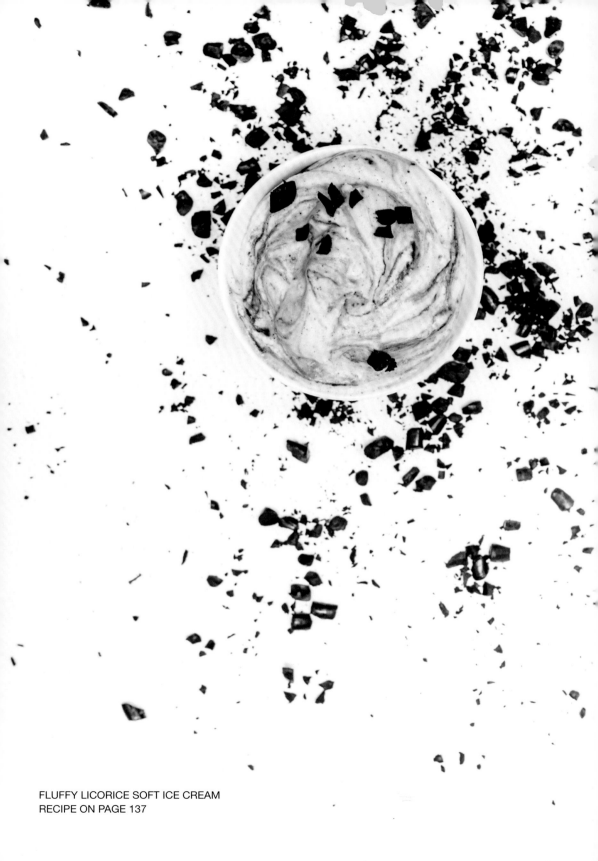

FLUFFY LICORICE SOFT ICE CREAM
RECIPE ON PAGE 137

BANANA SPLIT

BEAUTY BONUS NO. 43

Banana contains potassium, which is a regulator of the body's fluid balance and can contribute to reducing puffy eyes. Chocolate sauce is a liquid rejuvenation elixir with anti-wrinkle antioxidants from the raw cacao and immune-boosting fatty acids from coconut oil.

Raw banana split with chocolate sauce

This blessed creation is not just a marvel of deliciousness. It also earns so many beauty points that the beauty foodie in me is almost cross-eyed with excitement. With banana slices in the freezer, ice cream is never far away. In the blender, frozen banana slices are magically transformed into fluffy, soft ice cream. The recipe is for two people, but I can easily eat the whole thing on my own. The ice cream melts fast, so dive in as quick as you can.

2 SERVINGS
ICE CREAM
4 bananas, sliced and frozen
pinch of vanilla powder
1 tablespoon plant-based milk, if required
¼ cup raw cacao

RAW CHOCOLATE SAUCE
½ cup coconut oil
⅓ cup yacon syrup or coconut nectar
3–4 tablespoons raw cacao
1 teaspoon vanilla powder

TOPPING
toasted coconut chips
roasted almond chips
fresh berries (optional)

First make the sauce. Heat the coconut oil until it becomes liquid but not hot. Stir in the yacon syrup or coconut nectar, cacao, and vanilla to make a smooth sauce. Set aside.

Blend the bananas and vanilla in a high-speed blender to a soft ice cream consistency, adding a splash of milk if the blades have difficulty spinning. Divide half of the ice cream between 2 bowls. Add the cacao to the remaining ice cream in the blender and blend to make chocolate ice cream.

Scoop the chocolate ice cream into the bowls, drizzle with the chocolate sauce, and sprinkle with the toppings. Serve immediately—the ice cream melts quickly.

Chocolate caramel shortbread stix for a beauty fix

To hold these without messing up your fingers, leave the end of it undipped.

ABOUT 16 RECTANGLES
COOKIE DOUGH
1¾ cups coconut flour
3½ tablespoons maple syrup
½ teaspoon salt
⅓ cup coconut oil

TOPPING
½ cup coconut oil
⅓ cup almond or peanut butter
½ cup maple syrup
pinch of vanilla powder
½ teaspoon salt (optional if the nut butter is already salted)

CHOCOLATE COATING
½ cup coconut oil
½ cup maple syrup
1 cup raw cacao
1 teaspoon vanilla powder

Preheat the oven to 350°F. Line a rectangular baking pan with parchment paper. Mix together the coconut flour, syrup, and salt in a bowl until it becomes grainy. Stir the coconut oil until soft, then add to the coconut flour mixture and work together quickly into a clump. Press the dough into the prepared pan and bake in the middle of the oven for about 13 minutes, until golden at the edges. Let cool.

Melt the coconut oil for the topping in a saucepan, then stir together with the nut butter, syrup, vanilla, and salt until completely smooth. Pour the filling over the cooled shortbread, then put into the freezer. When the topping is firm, remove and cut into 16 rectangles.

To make the chocolate coating, melt the coconut oil in a saucepan until just liquid but not hot. Stir in the maple syrup, cacao, and vanilla until smooth. Dip the shortbreads into the chocolate, put onto a baking sheet lined with parchment paper, and let set in the refrigerator.

Nut-free raw chocolate balls

Choose gluten-free oats if you want gluten-free balls.

ABOUT 8 LARGE OR 16 SMALL BALLS
20 dates
½ cup strong, cold coffee
¼ cup raw cacao
¼ teaspoon vanilla powder
¼ teaspoon salt
2 tablespoons yacon syrup, maple syrup, or coconut nectar
3¾ cups rolled oats, plus extra if required
unsweetened dried coconut

Pit the dates, then process with the coffee, cacao, vanilla, salt, and syrup or nectar in a food processor. Put the oats into a large bowl, add the chocolate mixture, and work together into a soft dough. Add more oats if you want a drier mixture. Shape into balls, then roll in coconut. Store in the refrigerator.

Raw chocolate mousse

This mousse takes two minutes to make. The milk gives it a milk-chocolaty flavor and is optional if you prefer a darker chocolate flavor.

2–3 SERVINGS
2 avocados
3 tablespoons raw cacao
¼ cup yacon syrup or coconut nectar
1 tablespoon plant-based milk (optional)
1 teaspoon vanilla powder
1 tablespoon raw cacao nibs

Blend all the ingredients except the cacao nibs with a handheld blender until completely smooth. When you think the mousse is smooth, blend it some more. It should be as smooth as velvet. Top with the cacao nibs for extra crunch.

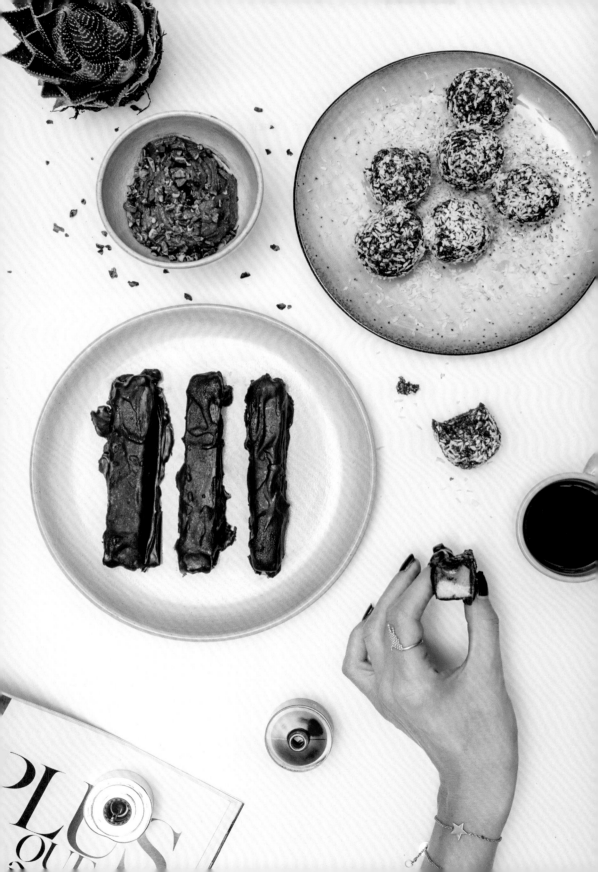

Vera's gingerbread balls with orange frosting

Ho ho ho, are there any nice children with Christmas wishes on their list? These gingerbread balls are a great Christmas gift to the skin, and taste like first-class gingerbread dough. The recipe came to me when my daughter Vera was craving gingerbread and I saw my chance to beauty-proof Christmas. Serve at a Christmas party, Advent celebration, or on Christmas Eve. Note: Don't have a pastry bag? Snip a hole in one corner of a regular plastic food or freezer bag.

ABOUT 8 LARGE OR 16 SMALL BALLS
20 dates
juice and finely grated zest of 1 orange
1 cup hazelnuts
1 cup almonds
2 teaspoons gingerbread spice

ORANGE FROSTING
1 cup cashew nuts
½ cup coconut oil
juice and finely grated zest of 1 orange
juice and finely grated zest of 1 lime
½ cup yacon syrup or coconut nectar
pinch of vanilla powder

TO DECORATE
walnuts

Soak the cashew nuts for the frosting in water for at least 2 hours, then drain well and rinse.

To make the frosting, stir the coconut oil until soft, then blend with the rest of the frosting ingredients in a high-speed blender until smooth. Stir in the orange and lime zest, reserving some orange zest to decorate. Put the mixture into a pastry bag and freeze for 10 minutes while making the balls.

Pit the dates, then soak in water. Drain, then process in a food processor with the orange juice and zest, hazelnuts, almonds, and spice until it makes a gooey paste. It's fine to keep some crunchy nut pieces in the mixture.

Roll into balls, then pipe a little frosting on each. Top with a walnut piece and some orange zest. Refrigerate until serving.

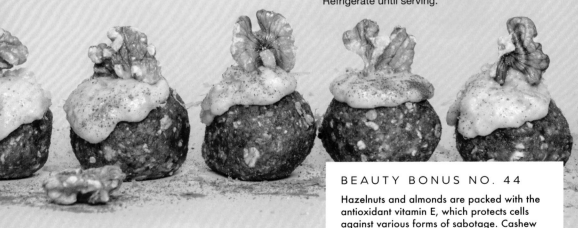

BEAUTY BONUS NO. 44

Hazelnuts and almonds are packed with the antioxidant vitamin E, which protects cells against various forms of sabotage. Cashew nuts are rich in iron, the alpha and omega of the body's oxygen transport system, which looks after hair and skin (anyone who's had brittle hair from iron deficiency can relate).

Fluffy licorice soft ice cream

This ice cream recipe came to me one evening when I had an acute craving for both licorice and ice cream. And what's better than licorice ice cream? Coconut cream is best when whipped with cold utensils, so toss the mixer beaters into the freezer as soon as you feel an ice cream craving coming on. If you don't have the patience to wait for the cream mixture to freeze to ice cream, it's just as good eaten right away—a fluffy, marshmallow-like licorice cloud without any shame. Raw licorice drops are available in well-stocked candy stores, health-food stores, and grocery stores.

2 SERVINGS
1 cup coconut cream
2 tablespoons coconut sugar
pinch of vanilla powder
2 teaspoons licorice powder, plus
    extra to taste
1 tablespoon raw licorice drops

Whisk the coconut cream, coconut sugar, and vanilla with a handheld electric mixer until fluffy. Fold in the licorice powder and whisk until combined. Add more licorice powder, if you want. Put into the freezer until firm. Using a mortar and pestle, crush the licorice drops into small pieces, then sprinkle on top before serving.

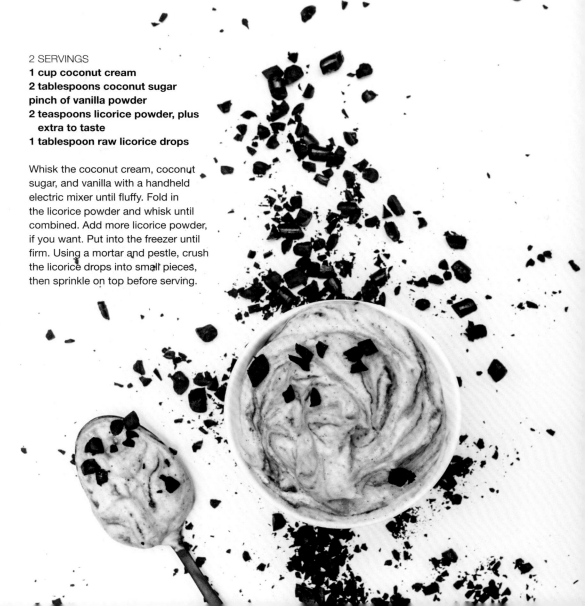

Glow-boosting ice cream pops

Magnum, move over. This is deliciousness on a stick. Ice cream pop molds can be found in hobby and kitchen stores. I use the Nicolas Vahé brand, available for purchase online. Vanilla ice cream is tasty as it is, but feel free to experiment with all kinds of flavors. Sometimes I make different flavors and build colorful layers in the molds. You can vary the ice cream with an infinite number of flavor combinations, coatings, and decorations. Here are my recipes for raw coatings with chocolate and caramel flavors, but if you're impatient, you can melt a fine baking chocolate with at least 85 percent cocoa solids and drizzle it over the ice cream. Roll the coated pops in crushed nuts, toasted coconut chips, or raw cacao nibs.

ABOUT 8 ICE CREAM POPS
ICE CREAM
2½ cups cashew nuts
1 cup coconut cream
½ cup yacon syrup or coconut nectar
1 teaspoon vanilla powder

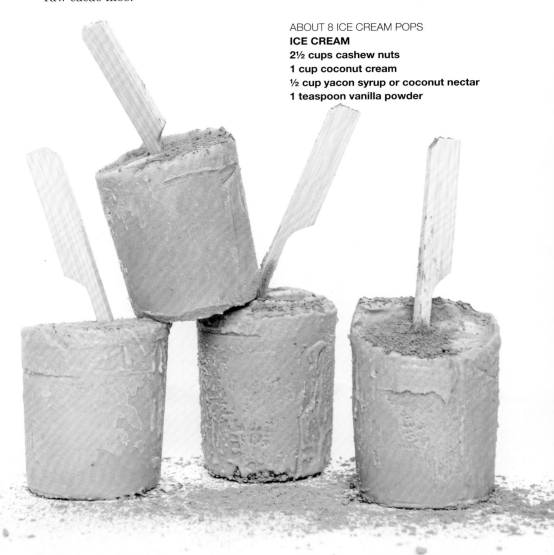

FLAVORINGS
LIME AND MATCHA
1 tablespoon matcha powder
juice of 2 limes
3 tablespoons extra sweetener

CHOCOLATE
3–4 tablespoons raw cacao

RASPBERRY
4 cups fresh or frozen raspberries

COATINGS
RAW CHOCOLATE
½ cup coconut oil
¼ cup raw cacao, plus extra to taste
1 teaspoon vanilla powder, plus extra to taste
⅓ cup yacon syrup or coconut nectar, plus
    extra to taste

RAW CARAMEL
½ cup coconut oil
1 tablespoon mesquite flour, plus extra to taste
1 teaspoon vanilla powder, plus extra to taste
⅓ cup yacon syrup or coconut nectar, plus
    extra to taste

To make the ice cream, soak the cashew nuts in water for about 2 hours. Drain, then rinse the nuts thoroughly in cold water and let drain. Blend the nuts in a high-speed blender with the coconut cream, syrup or nectar, and vanilla until smooth and fluffy.

Make your chosen flavoring and blend into the ice cream mixture until completely combined. If you want to use several flavorings, divide the ice cream mixture among several bowls and mix in the flavoring.

Pour the mixture into ice cream pop molds. Insert the sticks and put into the freezer for at least 4 hours.

To make the coatings, gently melt the coconut oil until just liquid, then let cool—it must not be so hot that the ice cream melts. Add the cacao, if making the chocolate coating, or the mesquite, if making the caramel coating, then stir in the vanilla and syrup or nectar with a fork until the coating is completely smooth. Taste and add more sweetener or cacao or mesquite to taste.

Remove the pops from the molds (rinse the outside of the mold quickly in hot water if you have difficulty loosening them). Dip the tip of each ice cream into the chocolate or caramel, or spread over the whole pop using a spatula.

Dip in crushed nuts, coconut, or whatever you want. Put the pops onto a plate lined with wax or parchment paper and put into the freezer to set.

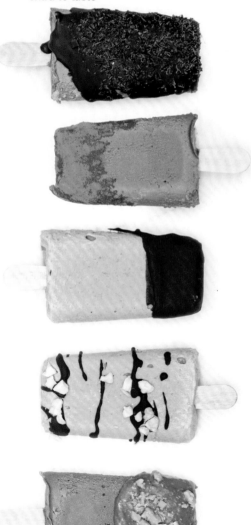

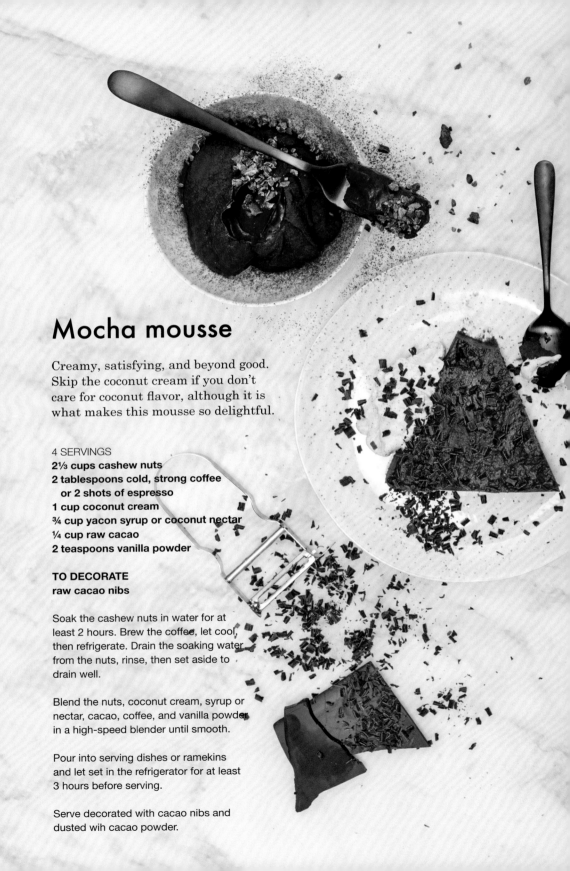

Mocha mousse

Creamy, satisfying, and beyond good.
Skip the coconut cream if you don't
care for coconut flavor, although it is
what makes this mousse so delightful.

4 SERVINGS
2⅓ cups cashew nuts
2 tablespoons cold, strong coffee
or 2 shots of espresso
1 cup coconut cream
¾ cup yacon syrup or coconut nectar
¼ cup raw cacao
2 teaspoons vanilla powder

TO DECORATE
raw cacao nibs

Soak the cashew nuts in water for at
least 2 hours. Brew the coffee, let cool,
then refrigerate. Drain the soaking water
from the nuts, rinse, then set aside to
drain well.

Blend the nuts, coconut cream, syrup or
nectar, cacao, coffee, and vanilla powder
in a high-speed blender until smooth.

Pour into serving dishes or ramekins
and let set in the refrigerator for at least
3 hours before serving.

Serve decorated with cacao nibs and
dusted wih cacao powder.

Boozy raw orange brownie cake

One New Year's Eve, we suddenly found ourselves without dessert when the gang's master chef became ill at the last minute. One of the girls suggested ice cream and berries, but I shouted: "Stop everything! It's New Year's Eve! We have to have chocolate!" So that afternoon I searched my pantry in a panic for stuff that I could quickly turn into a decadent dessert without getting my skin into trouble. We happened to have Cointreau, but Grand Marnier works just as well. If you want an alcohol-free cake, replace the booze with extra orange juice. Spend a little extra when selecting a fine baking chocolate for the icing—it should be something really luxurious and dark, and perhaps with an orange flavor, so that the resulting cake is as dark as sin and definitely not child friendly. A New Year's kiss will taste of orange liqueur and bittersweet midnight-dark chocolate.

4 SERVINGS
20 dates
¾ cup cashew nuts
3 tablespoons orange liqueur
juice of 1 orange
½ cup coconut oil
¼ cup raw cacao
1 tablespoon yacon syrup, maple syrup, or
   coconut nectar
1 teaspoon vanilla powder

CHOCOLATE ICING
5¼ oz bittersweet chocolate, at least
   70 percent cocoa solids
1 tablespoon grated orange zest

TO DECORATE
¼ cup grated bittersweet chocolate, at least
   70 percent cocoa solids

TO SERVE
Coconut Whipped Cream (see recipe on
   page 125)

Pit the dates, then put into a bowl with the cashew nuts and pour over the liqueur and orange juice. Let soak for at least 1 hour.

Transfer the dates, nuts, and soaking liquid to a food processor and blend together with the coconut oil, cacao, syrup or nectar, and vanilla powder until smooth and gooey. Press into a baking pan lined with plastic wrap (place the overhanging plastic wrap on top of the batter when pressing into the pan to avoid sticking). Put into the freezer until firm.

When the cake has set, melt the chocolate for the icing in a microwave or in a heatproof bowl set over a saucepan of simmering water. Pour the chocolate over the cake. Sprinkle with the orange zest and put into the refrigerator until set. Sprinkle the grated chocolate over the cake before serving and serve with Coconut Whipped Cream.

BEAUTY BONUS NO. 45

Dates are small gold mines of vitamins, fiber, and minerals. Yes, they are sugar bombs, but the other ingredients reduce the overall glycemic load of the cake.

Pretty-in-pink strawberry "cheesecake" on a lemon and coconut layer

This "My Little Pony" pink cake tastes like summer and charms the skin. If it's not a dream, I don't know what is. Organic strawberries provide maximum beauty.

1 LARGE OR 2 SMALL "CHEESECAKES"

LEMON AND COCONUT LAYER
10 dates
3 tablespoons coconut oil
juice and finely grated zest of 1 lemon
1½ cups unsweetened dried coconut

STRAWBERRY FILLING
3 cups cashew nuts
½ cup coconut oil
3¼ cups strawberries, defrosted if frozen
1 cup coconut nectar
1 teaspoon vanilla powder

STRAWBERRY FROSTING
1¼ cups strawberries, defrosted if frozen
¼ cup coconut oil
¼ cup coconut nectar

TO DECORATE
toasted coconut chips
fresh strawberries (optional)

Soak the cashew nuts for the filling in cold water for about 4 hours.

To make the coconut layer, pit the dates, then coarsely chop them. Gently melt the coconut oil in a saucepan. Blend the dates, lemon juice and zest, dried coconut, and melted coconut oil in a high-speed blender to make a doughy paste. Press the dough into a single layer in 1 large or 2 small springform cake pans. Put into the freezer.

Drain the cashew nuts, then rinse and let drain in a strainer. Gently melt the coconut oil for the filling in a saucepan. Blend the nuts and melted coconut oil with the strawberries, coconut nectar, and vanilla in a high-speed blender. Pour this cheeselike mixture over the coconut layer(s) and return to the freezer.

To make the frosting, blend the strawberries, coconut oil, and coconut nectar with a hand-held blender until smooth. Pour over the cheesecakes, then return to the freezer. Defrost in the refrigerator for 1 hour before serving, decorated with coconut chips and strawberries, if you want.

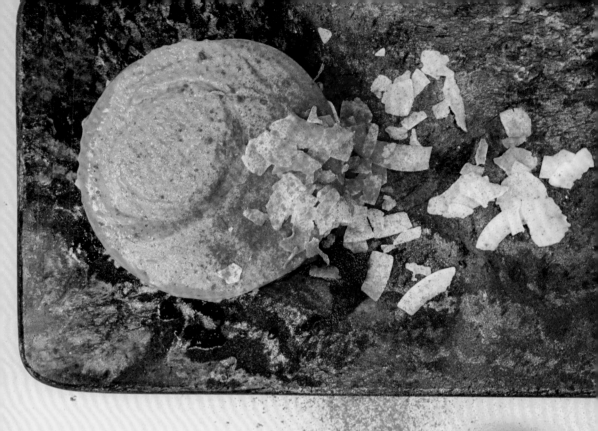

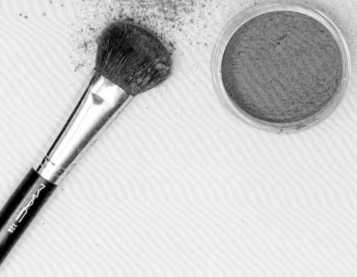

BEAUTY BONUS NO. 46

A handful of strawberries contains more collagen-building vitamin C than an entire orange. The ellagic acid provides UV protection, making strawberries a summer must (of course, in combination with a sunscreen of SPF 30 plus).

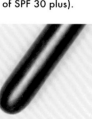

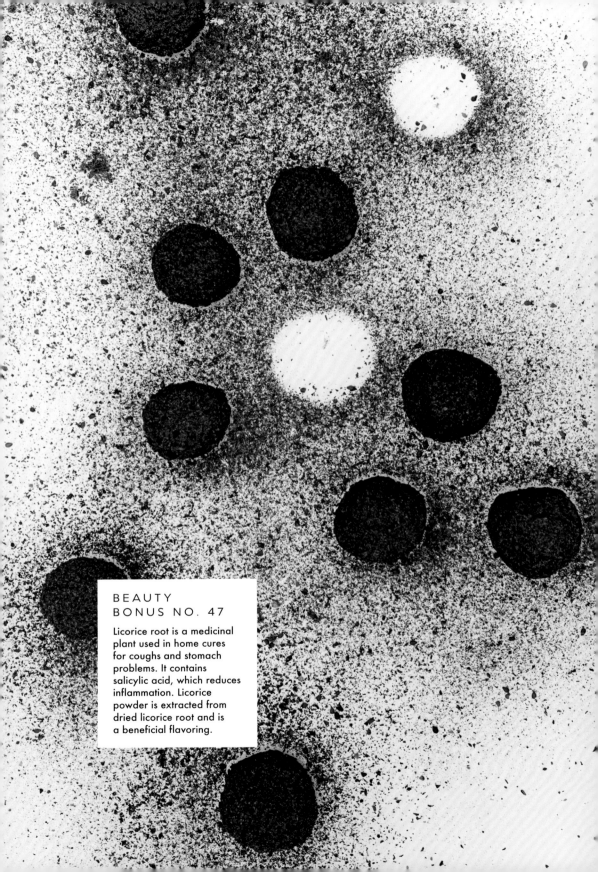

BEAUTY
BONUS NO. 47

Licorice root is a medicinal
plant used in home cures
for coughs and stomach
problems. It contains
salicylic acid, which reduces
inflammation. Licorice
powder is extracted from
dried licorice root and is
a beneficial flavoring.

Salted licorice truffles

Next to chocolate, licorice is the best. My favorite licorice treat is Salta Katten—The Salty Cat—a Scandinavian chewy candy that is sold in cute retro boxes. In homage, I created these salty licorice bombs, which fill the licorice lover and beauty foodie in me with happiness. If you get slightly larger dates, such as medjool, around 10 dates will be enough. Licorice powder can be found in health-food stores or online.

ABOUT 18 TRUFFLES
¾ cup cashew nuts
⅔ cup black sesame seeds,
    plus ¼ cup for rolling the truffles
15 dates
4 teaspoons licorice powder,
    plus 1 teaspoon for rolling the truffles
¼ cup yacon syrup or coconut nectar

Process the cashew nuts and sesame seeds in a food processor until they form a coarse meal. Pit the dates, add to the processor, and process until the mixture is grainy. Add the licorice powder and syrup or nectar and blend to a smooth, glossy paste.

Shape into balls, then roll in a mixture of sesame seeds and a little extra licorice powder. Store in the refrigerator.

Inner glow chocolate caramel cake

This cake tastes like Dumle, a brand of irresistibly gooey chocolate-covered toffees that is as cult as a candy can get in Sweden. The caramel flavor comes from mesquite flour, which may require a little research to find, but I promise it's worth the effort. It gives a creamy caramel taste without causing any trouble for your blood sugar. Plan B is to make a caramel from dates (see opposite), and, of course, there's nothing wrong with that either.

ABOUT 9 PIECES
1 tablespoon coconut oil
2½ cups rolled oats
1¼ cup cashew nuts
3–4 tablespoons raw cacao
1 teaspoon vanilla powder
¼ cup cold, strong coffee
⅓ cup yacon syrup or coconut nectar

SALTED CARAMEL
½ cup coconut oil
⅓ cup yacon syrup or coconut nectar
1 tablespoon mesquite flour
1 teaspoon vanilla powder
½ teaspoon sea salt flakes

CHOCOLATE ICING
1¾ oz good-quality bittersweet chocolate,
  at least 85 percent cocoa solids

Line a dish, about 6 × 6 inches, with plastic wrap (I often use a plastic storage container as a mold). Melt the coconut oil until it becomes just liquid. Process the oats and cashew nuts into a fine flour in a food processor. Transfer to a bowl. Stir in the cocoa, vanilla, coffee, syrup or nectar, and melted coconut oil. Stir together, then press the dough into the prepared dish. Put into the freezer.

Gently melt the coconut oil for the caramel in a saucepan, then let cool slightly until still liquid but not hot. Stir together the melted coconut oil, syrup or nectar, mesquite, vanilla, and salt until completely smooth. Remove the oat layer from the freezer and spread the caramel over it evenly. Return to the freezer.

Melt the chocolate for the icing in a microwave or in a heatproof bowl set over a saucepan of simmering water, then let cool a little. Remove the slightly hardened cake from the freezer and pour over the chocolate. Return to the freezer until firm. Transfer the cake to the refrigerator for at least 1 hour before serving.

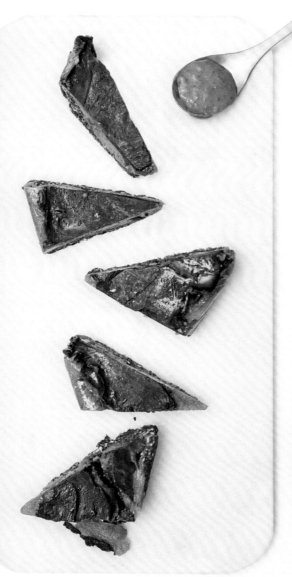

Plan B caramel made from dates

Use large, unpitted dates, such as medjool.

2 cups water
20 dates
a pinch of sea salt flakes, plus more
** to taste**
1 teaspoon vanilla powder

Heat the measured water. Pit the dates, then soak in the water for 10 minutes. Pour off the soaking water, but reserve it. Put the dates into a small food processor with the salt and vanilla. If the blades have difficulty spinning, add a splash of the soaking water, but only up to 1 tablespoon at a time—too much water will destroy the caramel consistency. Add more salt to taste.

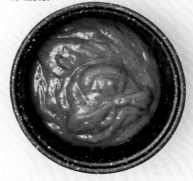

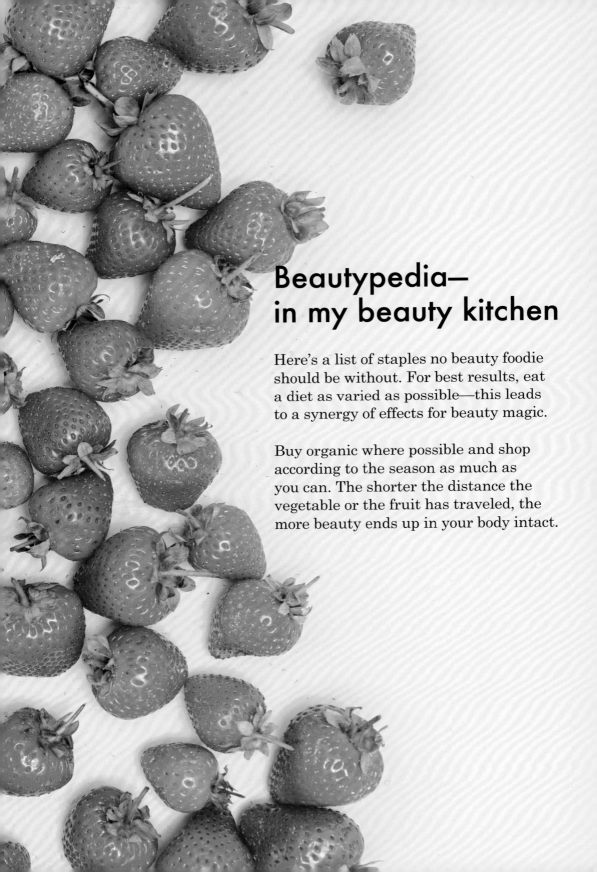

Beautypedia—
in my beauty kitchen

Here's a list of staples no beauty foodie
should be without. For best results, eat
a diet as varied as possible—this leads
to a synergy of effects for beauty magic.

Buy organic where possible and shop
according to the season as much as
you can. The shorter the distance the
vegetable or the fruit has traveled, the
more beauty ends up in your body intact.

ALGAE—jewels of the sea

Spirulina, wakame, hijiki, nori, arame, dulse, kombu, or chlorella—edible algae are bursting with beauty-boosting trace minerals and the best fatty acid, omega-3. They are also a really environmentally friendly source of protein. In the future, we will all be powered by algae, mark my words! Algae have a high content of iodine, which has effects on the metabolism, so if you have a thyroid disorder, you should check with your physician before adding algae to your daily menu.

ALMONDS—free radical vacuum cleaner

No wrinkles from here on out! Almonds boast one of nature's highest contents of vitamin E, which protects our valuable cell membranes. Think of vitamin E as the police officer that rounds up free radicals. These helpful nuts are also rich in magnesium. Almond milk is a top dairy alternative—some studies indicate that dairy can trigger existing acne problems, so plant-based milks, such as almond, can be handy.

APPLE—beauty soldier of the fruit basket

The apple is already honored with granting knowledge, but I want to give it a new title—beauty food. Apple peel contains the antioxidant quercetin, which strengthens the skin's natural protection against free radicals. Red apples can take pride in their flavonoid anthocyanins. An apple a day keeps wrinkles at bay!

ASPARAGUS—eraser of sleepless nights

A top source of folic acid, which is needed for the body to produce red blood cells. Contains vitamin E (which protects the skin's tightness), the mildly acting amino acid asparagine, and vitamin K, which strengthens the blood vessels and can reduce dark circles around the eyes.

AVOCADO—moisturizer for the inside

Too bad skin was denied this amazing beauty fruit during the fat-fearing 1980s and 90s. And this, in combo with those decades' obsession with sunbathing—avocado and a sensible sunscreen could have avoided a lot of roast-beef cleavage! If, with a knife held to my throat, I had to choose only five beauty foods to eat for the rest of my life, avocado would be on the list. Pursuit of the perfect avocado is as nerve-racking as Russian roulette, but once on the plate, it offers a bonanza of monounsaturated fats, which moisturize the skin from the inside; provides satisfying fiber and important antioxidants, including skin-friendly vitamin E to protect against UV damage; and keeps your skin elastic and glowing.

BANANA—stop sign for eye bags

Bananas are a power pack of mood- and beauty-enhancing vitamins, minerals, and fiber. Potassium controls the body's fluid balance, which means smaller bags under the eyes, and silicon waves its magic wand over hair and nails. The banana also feeds good bacteria in the stomach. The best are unripe, green bananas.

BEANS—little pods of beauty

With its economical connection to frankfurters, the bean lives a quiet existence far from glamor and beauty salons. But beans are true beauty packages, containing supportive proteins; beauty-boosting minerals and vitamins; and slow-release carbohydrates and fibers, which counteract blood-sugar peaks and keep you feeling fuller for longer. They are also environmentally friendly and cheap.

BLUEBERRIES—nature's rejuvenation pills

You know those silly T-shirts that occasionally show up on large men: "This body was built by beer"? On my T-shirt, it would say that my body, or at least my skin, was built by blueberries. At the dental hygienist, I am known as "the one with blueberry stains on her teeth." But blueberries are so good, as well as beautiful. The color comes from the anthocyanin pigment, an antioxidant that is pure rocket fuel for resilient, elastic skin that can better withstand UV damage and attacks from beauty-sabotaging free radicals. Also, blueberries contain beauty vitamins C and E, and stomach-friendly fiber.

BROCCOLI—first aid for dark circles

If any vegetable is entitled to claim the title "superfood," broccoli is definitely a hot candidate. The beautiful leafy green bouquets contain high levels of vitamin K to boost the circulation, strengthen the capillaries, and fight dark circles under the eyes (vitamin K is often used in eye creams). This beauty cocktail also includes skin-tightening vitamins C and A, carotenoids, folate, calcium, and fiber. In addition, there are sulfur-containing phytochemicals that can inhibit stress-related inflammations and stimulate enzymes that help the body's natural cleansing system to get rid of harmful substances. Forget the expensive detox powder and eat some extra broccoli instead. In the United States, a bunch of scientists have found that, in animal studies, broccoli can also help the skin to repair sun damage.

BROWN RICE—the fabulous grain

As you can see in my recipes, I use short-grain brown rice in everything from salads to bowls.

During my four years in Tokyo, I ate brown rice (genmai) every day and have never felt better. Unpolished, short-grain brown rice is high in fiber, the B vitamins, and minerals, all of which contribute to smooth skin and beautiful hair and nails. It also contains ceramides, a type of lipid (fat) that is naturally present in the skin, which contributes to well-functioning skin.

BUCKWHEAT—gluten-free and skin friendly

Buckwheat is not a wheat but a plant packed with beauty nutrients. The phytonutrient rutin reduces wrinkle-inducing advanced glycation end products (AGEs; see Beauty Saboteurs on page 19). Buckwheat is also a good source of vitamins, minerals, slow-release carbohydrates, and essential amino acids. Gluten-free pancakes and waffles made with buckwheat are scrumptious for the inside and outside.

CACAO (RAW) AND CACAO NIBS—better than Botox

It's no news that dark chocolate with at least 70 percent cocoa solids is health friendly, but for the skin, it's the cacao itself that's the hero. The potent flavonoid (an antioxidant übergroup) epicatechin prevents the appearance of wrinkles. Raw cacao also has a higher value oxygen radical absorbance capacity (ORAC; that is, antioxidant effect) than goji berries, blueberries, and green tea. Cacao is also exciting because it increases neurotransmitters, such as serotonin and endorphins, in the brain. In addition, cacao contains magnesium—nature's own chill pill. In order for us to experience these benefits and be smoother, happier, and calmer, untreated (that is, raw) cacao is required. Choose raw cacao nibs or raw chocolate containing at least 70 percent cocoa solids. For PMS, in particular, I prescribe a lot of extra chocolate!

CARROT—built-in SPF

Beta-carotene is converted into vitamin A in the liver, which helps the body to repair aging skin tissue and keep up collagen production. It also boosts the skin's defense against sun damage, which means not only protection against cell damage but also a smoother, deeper, and more durable tan. However, sun protection with factor 30 is still a nonnegotiable must. Also contains vitamin C and biotin, which is important for the hair.

CAULIFLOWER—wrinkle-fighting bouquet

Cruciferous vegetables, such as broccoli and other types of cabbage, including cauliflower, contain an exciting phytochemical called sulforaphane—a powerful antioxidant that counteracts premature aging. Cauliflower is rich in vitamin A, folic acid, potassium, and vitamin C, which are required for the formation of collagen.

CELERY—hair booster with crunch

Popular among some dieters for its water-loss effect. However, it's not just the bladder but also your hair follicles that can benefit from a boost of celery, because it contains silicon, a traditional ingredient in dietary supplements for the hair. Vitamin C accelerates collagen synthesis.

CHIA SEEDS—vegan-friendly omega-3

These seeds are 20 percent of the beauty kitchen's favorite, omega-3 fatty acid, which can reduce inflammation and protect against various types of aging. It's a complete protein with all the building blocks that skin, hair, and nails need. It also provides loads of dietary fiber, which keeps the stomach balanced and flat.

COCONUT OIL—the energy kick

Half of the fat in coconut oil comes from lauric acid. This acid burns quickly, which has made it popular with dieters—especially those in the low-carbohydrate camp. Lauric acid and caprylic acid are also present in breast milk and are attributed with certain viral, fungal, bactericidal, and antioxidant effects. Unlike cold-pressed olive and canola oil, coconut oil tolerates high temperatures. As a beauty foodie, omega-3 is my favorite fat companion, but in sweet things and at high temperatures, coconut oil is the best choice.

CUCUMBER—cooling thirst extinguisher

Comprises 95 percent water, which is the basic prerequisite for moisture-saturated, bright skin. As a beauty foodie, I also dig that the cucumber skin has a high silicon content, which keeps collagen and connective tissue in top shape and strengthens your hair. Always buy organic so you can eat the skin.

DATES—sweetie with a beauty bonus

Desserts were my entrance ticket into the raw food world, and I swallowed uncritically and wholeheartedly the "dessert for dinner" argument, but then I found out there are all kinds of raw food dishes—however, fermented cabbage and raw, shredded broccoli don't sound nearly as appealing. Excessive intake of raw desserts is, of course, not recommended, but from time to time, as a treat, dates are a nice beauty friend that contain vitamin C and a good array of the B vitamins, as well as minerals, such as iron, magnesium, and potassium, which inhibits fluid retention (so long, puffy eyes!).

EGGPLANT—protective beauty

The dark beauty of the eggplant's skin is not just ideal for a glamorous lipstick (Chanel Rouge Allure in shade 109 Rouge Noir is pure perfection) or nail varnish (OPI Lincoln Park After Dark is always in my refrigerator). No, the color indicates the presence of superantioxidant and phytochemical anthocyanins, which also give blueberries, plums, cranberries, and black currants their elegant hue. It's the anthocyanin nasunin that particularly interests us skin junkies; it is a potent antioxidant that can protect skin cells from being damaged by free radicals. The flesh is rich in dietary fiber and the B vitamins, which gives you glossy hair and strong nails.

EGGS—an edible hair treatment

Does your hair feel lifeless? Four eggs a week will strengthen your hair and give it a new glow in just a few weeks. Eggs contain sulfur—which is an important component of skin, hair, nails, and body tissues—and loads of complete protein that builds both skin and hair. The egg is also packed with vitamins A and D. When I feel that my hair is sad and brittle, I cook pancakes and waffles. Choose omega-3-enriched eggs for extra beauty points.

GINGER—anti-inflammatory superstar

This knotty root not only relieves stomach ache, nausea, muscle aches, and general aches, it is also healing to the skin. Packed with anti-inflammatory substances, ginger can relieve conditions, such as redness and acne problems, and the substance gingerol counteracts the breakdown of the protein elastin in the skin. Blood circulation gets a heavy boost, which points to ginger's potential for stimulating hair growth.

GOJI—much-hyped antiaging berries

The amino acid glutamine stimulates the body's production of human growth hormone (HGH), which helps the skin to maintain its wow factor. Contains carotenoids, which protect the skin against sun damage; important amino acids; fiber; and antioxidants that protect the DNA. Here, it's important to buy only organic—goji berries from China are often sprayed, and we don't want that in our beauty routine.

GREEN TEA AND MATCHA—Eastern wisdom for body and soul

When I was a teenager experiencing severe eczema, my dad lived in Hong Kong and worked in the medicine industry. Dad's Chinese physician companions provided me with green tea, which they said could relieve my skin problems. The effect on eczema hasn't been scientifically proven, nor has the alleged effect on acne, but we know that green tea contains polyphenols that protect against free radicals. Matcha green tea is the powdered leaves of tea plants grown in shade, so the concentration of beauty nutrition becomes higher. Buy organic.

HEMP SEEDS—perfect balance of fat

Containing all essential amino acids, hemp seeds have an optimal balance between the omega-3 and omega-6 fatty acids, and, as studies indicate, they can ease dry and eczema-prone skin. They also contain the fatty acid gamma linolenic acid (GLA), which balances volatile hormones. Thank you, says the PMS monster.

KALE—supermodel favorite

Full of vitamin K, which strengthens blood vessels and makes sure that blood circulation works as it should. With good circulation follows healthy skin and a healthier look when dark circles under the eyes start to decrease. Kale is also host to the mega-antioxidants lutein and zeaxanthin, which belong to the carotenoid group, and act as a kind of inner sunscreen (but don't skip your sunscreen lotion). A little unexpectedly, kale also contains the skin- and hair-loving omega-3 fatty acid. In addition, cell renewal is stimulated, which means that fresh, glowing skin cells will soon rise to the surface. A must in every respectable beauty kitchen.

KIWIFRUIT—beauty-maximizing sleeping pill

A small kiwi contains a whole day's vitamin C requirement, which we know is the alpha and omega of collagen formation (the skin's "padding") and protects against beauty-sabotaging free radicals. Kiwis can also protect our DNA from free radical attacks and, according to some studies, improve beauty sleep. As a constant insomniac, I thank and bow to the kiwi, and like to have a kiwi as a nightcap.

LEMON—sour collagen jump-starter

In interviews about their beauty habits, models and celebrities often tell you to start the day with lemon squeezed into warm water to keep your stomach flat and skin in good condition (Beyoncé is said to be a fan of living for periods of time on a beauty tonic of lemon, maple syrup, and cayenne pepper). There are no proper scientific studies on lemon intake and acne, but many find that their acne lightens and that the skin becomes clearer when they regularly have some hot lemon in the morning. Try it for yourself (but use a straw so you don't damage the enamel on your teeth). From a beauty point of view, the high content of collagen-building vitamin C is the lemon's greatest ingredient. Antioxidants mop up beauty-destructive free radicals, strengthen the immune system, and produce tight, glowing skin that is better equipped to handle external threats. Vitamin C also helps the body to absorb iron from food.

LIME—skin-friendly charmer
Like its cousin the lemon, lime has a fabulous vitamin C content and, therefore, both immune- and skin-boosting effects. Use freely in cooking and smoothies, because vitamin C helps the body absorb iron. Besides, it's oh so good! Did someone say mojito?

LINGONBERRIES—Nordic youth protector
Contain the substance resveratrol, an antioxidant that also thrives in wine grapes (and, therefore, in wine) and is hailed as one of the secrets why the French are aging with such enviable grace. Google "the French Paradox." Lingonberries can be hard to find, but you can order them frozen online, or substitute with frozen cranberries (although extra sweetness might be needed if you use these).

LUCUMA—creamy caramel flavoring
The flesh of the South American lucuma fruit is rich in beta-carotene, vitamin B_3, and fibre, but its real USP is the creamy caramel flavor. Lucuma is dried and milled into a powder that is sweet and caramel-like—the perfect flavoring for smoothies or raw ice cream.

MANGO—yellow gold
A yellow festival of skin-boosting vitamins! Beta-carotene, the yellow pigment that's converted into vitamin A, and vitamin C are a dream combo to treat aging skin. They fire up cell renewal and encourage new, glowing skin cells. Vitamin C supports collagen synthesis, which gives cheeks the consistency of freshly risen dough (hmm, feels more beautiful than it sounds). Vitamins help the skin retain moisture so that it feels deliciously juicy. Beta-carotene also enhances the skin's natural protection against the sun's wrinkle-inducing rays.

MESQUITE FLOUR—beauty-proofed caramel sauce
This caramel-like nutrition cocktail is hard to find, but if you do find it, grab it! (You can use dates as a substitute in recipes.) A few teaspoons of mesquite mixed with yacon syrup and coconut oil beat any store-bought ice cream sauce (freeze the mixture for a while and you have a sticky caramel). It beauty bombs all it touches with magnesium, potassium, iron, zinc, dietary fiber, and the amino acid lysine, and controls blood sugar. Check for it online or in health-food stores. A bag will last for a long time. Do not confuse it with mesquite barbecue wood!

MINT—zen for stomach and skin
Crunching mint leaves is like pampering the intestine with a yin yoga class, and, as we know, a well-functioning digestive system is the alpha and omega for the skin. Use in smoothies, salads, and beverages.

MISO—probiotic rock star
A vessel loaded with beauty-giving bacteria! Our stomachs love fermented food, and fermented soybean paste is brimming with antiaging and immune-strengthening properties. And a happy stomach leads to happy skin. If I learned one thing during my years in Japan, it's the following: Miso performs miracles for the inside and outside every day. Recipes are found in the chapter My Japanese beauty kitchen on page 82.

MUSHROOMS—beauty-shielding umami bomb
These happy little brown caps contain inflammation-disrupting and cell-shielding nutrition, the B vitamins, and high levels of selenium, which protect the skin's elasticity. All fungi are rich in antioxidants. Shiitake is a traditional medicinal mushroom that's extra rich in mega-antioxidant ergothioneine.

OATS—nature's gift to hair
In these stressful times, hair loss and/or premature hair loss is a common disease. The hair is, after all, the last priority of the body when it comes to nourishment, and if we are stressed or sick, the nutrition is distributed to more needy organs. One of the most common questions I get asked as a beauty editor is on hair loss and I always advise people to eat more oats. It contains a supercocktail of the B vitamins, magnesium, iron, and zinc, all of which are essential to the hair's health and color. Chocolate balls, oatmeal, or overnight oats are a gift to your hair, especially if combined with dietary supplements containing silicon, zinc, and biotin when feeling stressed.

OLIVE OIL—barrier against external beauty saboteurs
The Mediterranean's worst-kept health secret, olive oil has anti-inflammatory properties and vitamin E that protects the cell membranes and, together with vitamin C, creates a barrier against external beauty saboteurs. Use cold-pressed extra virgin olive oil, but avoid heating it because the nutrients are destroyed.

ONION—cheapest beauty investment
Many members of the onion family (white and red onion, garlic, leek, chives, scallions, and so on) are staples in the beauty kitchen.

Anti-inflammatory, cleansing effects build barriers against both pimples and fine lines, while flavonoids produce sky-high antioxidant activity. My stomach doesn't handle raw onion well, but cooked usually is fine. Scallions and leeks are easier on the stomach.

PEPPERS—fiesta for the skin
Of the bell peppers, the red ones are extremely rich in collagen-building vitamin C and the carotenoid lycopene. Yellow bell peppers also contain a good nutritional value, but the poor green ones aren't that interesting. Chili peppers are anti-inflammatory and boost the oh-so-important blood circulation.

PINEAPPLE—six-pack maker
Pineapple is stuffed with dietary fiber that boosts the ultra-important beauty digestion, but it also contains the bromelain enzyme that helps the breakdown of protein (hence the terrible sticky feeling in the throat when one happens to eat unripe pineapple). It is, therefore, known as the fruit that gives you a flat stomach. Rich in collagen-forming vitamin C, as well as magnesium and copper, which play a role in keeping graying hair at bay.

POMEGRANATE—ruby red skin love
Pomegranate seeds are probably the most beautiful things you can decorate a salad or a cake with. These small seeds deliver ellagic acid, which works against inflammation and the collapse of collagen. The seeds also help the blood to flow freely, bringing oxygen and nutrition to cells much more quickly.

PUMPKIN SEEDS—fighter of pimples and gray hairs
My favorite seed in all categories. Pumpkin seeds are nature's most potent zinc bomb, and zinc deficiency is linked to both acne and gray hair. Amino acid tryptophan helps the body to produce the calming and tranquillizing hormone serotonin. Like any acne patient with a few gray hairs, some mild anxiety, and sleep problems, I crack open pumpkin seeds on a daily basis.

QUINOA—protein power
One of the few vegetarian sources that contains all essential amino acids and, therefore, is considered a complete protein. Anti-inflammatory phytochemicals, important antioxidants, and high fiber content that keep blood sugar levels stable give quinoa an obvious place on the beauty plate.

RADISH—peppery beauty bomb
A huge dose of anti-inflammatory substances makes the radish a little extra worth crunching for those who have inflammatory skin conditions, such as acne or eczema (this, of course, doesn't replace medical treatment). Large quantities of vitamin C in combo with the beauty minerals sulfur and silicon make the radish a first-class beauty food.

RASPBERRIES—the skin-shielding gorgeous berry
These berries contain an impressive set of antioxidants, including collagen-protecting vitamin C, anti-inflammatory anthocyanins, and ellagic acid, which protect the cells against oxidative stress. They also contain smaller amounts of biotin that boost the hair and nails.

RED BEETS—cheapest detox method
You've probably heard that beets are the best medicine against a hangover. It gives the liver an extra boost, and this cleansing is also felt in the skin, which together with the liver is our major cleansing device. The red pigment strengthens both the immune system and the cells. Some people feel that their acne improves thanks to beets or beet juice.

RED WINE—the French Paradox
Having a glass of red wine with dinner is actually a good thing for beauty. In the grape skins, there's the antioxidant resveratrol, which is credited with the well-being of the French—despite all that wine and cheese. Choose organic (untreated grapes) with low sugar content.

SALMON—face mask, hair treatment, and brain enhancer all in one
This oily fish is filled with omega-3, which is pure gold for beauty hunters! It also provides collagen and elastin, which make the skin smooth and full. Hair that grows from a healthy scalp is extremely bright and shiny. Selenium is a powerful antioxidant that protects against sun damage. The salmon-pink color comes from astaxanthin, a true superantioxidant. Eating oily fish three times a week is like a lightning bolt for beauty—but also for our beloved brains.

SEA BUCKTHORN—essential for dryness
A staple in Chinese medicine to treat dry skin and mucous membranes. Its secret is omega-7 fatty acid. The little yellow bombs are also packed with vitamins C and E and beta-carotene.

SESAME SEEDS—nutty super seed
Unhulled sesame seeds are rich in, among other things, vitamin E, omega-3, calcium, zinc, and iron, and, being chewed or ground to butter as tahini, releases all the benefits. I love tahini as a base in dressings, and sesame seeds as a

topping on almost everything. In Japan, black sesame seeds are ground with sea salt to make gomashio. Crazy good on rice and vegetables.

SPINACH—glow food deluxe

Words can hardly do these beautiful super-leaves justice. Vitamin A keeps cells on their toes and acts as a delete button for cell damage. In addition, vitamin A seems to have a balancing effect on sebum production and, therefore, mitigates acne. The hyped antioxidant glutathione protects and repairs our DNA and mitochondria (the cells' power plants), while chlorophyll oxygenates the blood. Of course, we shouldn't forget the iron, which transports oxygen to skin and hair. For the iron to be absorbed, you need vitamin C, so squeeze some lemon over the leaves or blend a smoothie containing spinach and lime or lemon.

SPROUTS AND MICROGREENS—budding life

There's something touching about these tiny sprouts exploring this big world. Consume these and you'll receive a hefty dose of beauty with vitamins and enzymes that cells easily absorb. I'm not domesticated enough to grow my own sprouts, but I shop for alfalfa sprouts, mung bean sprouts, sunflower sprouts, red beet sprouts (adorably beautiful), or whatever else I can get my hands on.

STRAWBERRIES—wrinkle inhibitor

Who knew that a midsummer party is also a mini spa for the skin? That benefit is possibly outweighed by X number of shots of schnapps, but still. Each strawberry contains a wallop of vitamin C, which protects and builds collagen. A fistful of berries provides more vitamin C than an entire orange. They also contain ellagic acid, which helps cells ward away pimples, and manganese, which protects the cells' own power plants—mitochondria.

SWEET POTATO—first-class skin repairer

There's no ice cream van in Japan. Instead, there is a sweet potato van—no wonder that the Japanese have geisha-smooth skin. Sweet potatoes are stuffed with antioxidant beta-carotene, which the body turns into skin-repairing vitamin A. An injection of vitamins A and C makes sure that cell renewal is ticking like a Swiss clock.

TOMATO—beauty insurance

The red pigment lycopene is an extremely powerful antioxidant that erects a barrier against external beauty invaders. Free radicals, sun, inflammation, stress, or pollution—lycopene to the rescue! Maximum beautification is achieved when tomato is cooked and eaten with a little oil (Italian evening = beauty party). Even a simple tomato paste works well.

TURMERIC—all-round beauty booster

A must in the beauty kitchen! Like ginger, turmeric is a powerful anti-inflammatory, which can help skin conditions, such as acne, eczema, psoriasis, and rosacea. Curcumin, a substance in turmeric, is a lively antioxidant that sets up a shield against fine lines and wrinkles and stimulates collagen formation. It also aids the body's natural cleansing so that glow killers are wiped out, and it increases blood circulation so that all the delicious nutrition tours the body and goes straight to skin cells. Use fresh or dried. Also available as a supplement.

WALNUT—smart hydrator

One of the few foods from the plant kingdom containing skin-enhancing omega-3 in the form of alpha-linolenic acid (ALA). A small handful of walnuts a day helps keep skin moisture levels up during the winter. Also rich in antioxidants.

WATERMELON—beach season's savior

A summer without watermelon is unthinkable. Being a perfect combination of water and the beauty vitamins A and C makes watermelon a winner. The red color comes from lycopene, which protects the skin from sunburn (of course, this also requires a good sunscreen with at least SPF 30 as well). Lightly frozen watermelon slices are moisturizer in a tasty sorbet form.

YACON SYRUP—beauty-proofed sweetener

There are probably a lot of you who read my dessert recipes and wonder what this ever-present yacon syrup is. And yes, it's difficult to get hold of, but it can be found in well-stocked health-food stores and online. Yacon syrup is a liquid sweetener that has a low impact on blood sugar, which is gold from a beauty perspective. The syrup is extracted from the yacon root and tastes like a mixture of caramel and raisins. Almost 50 percent of its composition is the carbohydrate inulin, which is not absorbed by the body but which acts like a prebiotic and feeds good gastric bacteria. If you can't find yacon syrup, coconut nectar is a good option, preferable to agave.

ZUCCHINI—beauty hunter's spaghetti

Courgetti, or zucchini spaghetti—dear children have many names—this beauty-friendly alternative to pasta won't give your blood sugar a roller-coaster ride. The nutritional density is low, but a decent "pasta serving" will yield vitamin C and even a little hair-boosting folic acid.

DO SOME INGREDIENTS SEEM A LITTLE ODD?

Yacon, mesquite, lucuma, miso . . .
I understand that some ingredients
in the beauty food kitchen can be
a little difficult to get hold of, but
once you have them in your pantry,
you will never want to be without
them again. I promise! They're
the kitchen pantry's equivalent to
French pharmacist creams and hard-
to-find K-Beauty cult products. Once
in place, they raise your beauty
kitchen to new levels. Most can be
found online.

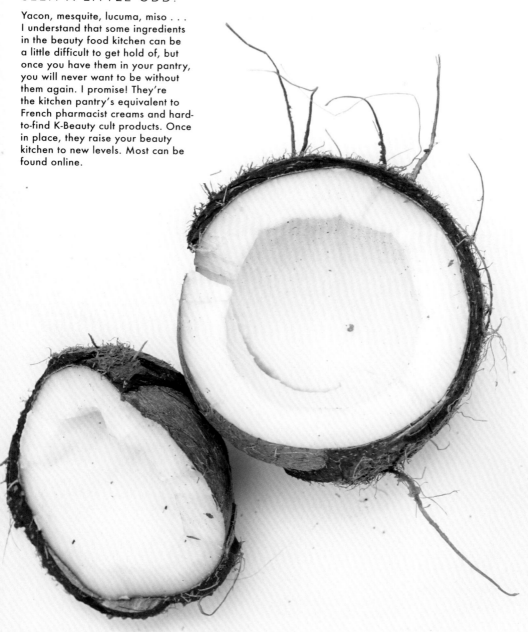

Beauty food phrasebook— your glossary in the beauty kitchen

AMINO ACIDS

Protein is the body's building block that repairs all tissues (including skin, hair, and nails), regulates hormone processes, builds muscle, and does a lot of other important things in the body. Amino acids are, in turn, the building blocks of protein. There are about 20 types altogether, of which 9 are called essential amino acids, which the body alone cannot produce. These can be created only by eating the right foods. Fish, eggs, plain yogurt, and quark are some of the best food sources of beauty-building amino acids. If you're vegan, so-called complete protein can be obtained from, among other things, tofu, edamame (green soybeans), lentils/beans (preferably in a brown rice combo to be full), quinoa, and buckwheat. Go protein!

ANTIOXIDANTS

This group has the nickname "nature's own antirusting agents" and is an umbrella term for nutritional components that counteract oxidation. Antioxidants neutralize oxygen molecules that have lost an electron and, therefore, become a beauty-absorbing free radical that irradiates around the cells in search of a new "tail." The antioxidants' Zen-like effect on the free radicals and so-called oxidative stress in the body gives them a beauty food place of honor. Most of those under the antioxidant umbrella contain phytochemicals (see opposite) and vitamins. The intensity of antioxidant activity in a raw material is measured using the oxygen radical absorbance capacity (ORAC) scale.

DIETARY FIBER

Keeps us full, builds up the bacterial flora of the stomach, and stabilizes blood sugar. From the beauty point of view, so-called soluble dietary fiber gets an extra gold star because it forms a gel around food as it travels through the body, thus stopping the beauty-sabotaging ups and downs of fluctuating blood sugar levels. Soluble dietary fiber is in vegetables, fruits, oats, berries, and seeds, such as flax, chia, and psyllium.

ENZYMES

Enzymes jump-start bodily functions and responses, and make sure they are operating as they should. Important for digestion, they ensure that the body can make good use of all the wonderful beauty nutrition it has absorbed. Fruit enzymes are also a VIP in peel products.

FATTY ACIDS

Help the body to function normally, produce hormones, and absorb fat-soluble beauty vitamins, such as A, D, E, and K. There are different types of fatty acid that help the skin to bathe in glow from the inside out. Beauty foodies are especially interested in omega-3 from fatty fish, algae, and polyunsaturated fatty acids. Avocado, nuts (especially walnuts), seeds, and cold-pressed oils, such as coconut, flaxseed, or olive, are fantastic beauty foods and have an automatic place in the beauty kitchen.

FREE RADICALS

The beauty criminal is the free radical, which is naturally formed by the body when the oxygen we breathe oxidizes, but also through lifestyle-related factors, such as UV radiation, sugar, some drugs, stress, and cigarette smoke. Free radicals are reactive acid molecules lacking an electron. They irradiate and emit electrons from cells in the body to create a domino effect. So-called oxidative stress occurs, and in a slightly oversimplified way, it could be said that the body is rusting from within. The best protection is antioxidants. Note: In medicine, current understanding about free radicals vs. antioxidants is being reexamined, and it doesn't seem to be as black and white as once thought. But from a beauty point of view, we should padlock the doors of Free Radical & Co.

MINERALS

This happy gang from the periodic table is important for keeping skin, hair, and nails in top shape. Zinc, magnesium, copper, iron, selenium, sulfur, iodine, and copper are some of the beauty minerals we obtain from our food. Sometimes food is not enough, and iron deficiency is especially common among us ladies, but it can be checked with a simple blood sample and adjusted with a supplement.

PHYTOCHEMICALS/PHYTONUTRIENTS

Nature's own immune system, made up of all the wonderful shades of the rainbow. These color-rich components protect the world's inhabitants from external stresses, UV rays, and diseases, and each color fulfills a purpose. Humans can benefit from the phytochemicals' protection against everyday beauty saboteurs. They often work in synergy and reinforce each other, so make a rainbow on your plate as often as possible. At least three colors create a beauty bomb. A large group of phytochemicals has a chemical structure called polyphenol, which is linked to a wide range of health benefits. Phytochemicals often have an antioxidative function. Some phytotypes, as listed below, are extraordinary dynamite for us beauty foodies:

Anthocyanins

These pigments are found in beautiful things, such as blueberries, cranberries, red cabbage, and plums, and protect the DNA in our cells whilst boosting the skin's elasticity.

Curcumin

This is turmeric's most hyped component, and contributes to its status as one of the most anti-inflammatory spices.

Carotenoids

Yellow-red pigments are appreciated in the beauty kitchen for their ability to protect cells against sun damage. These include beta-carotene (vitamin A precursor, found in carrots, sweet potatoes, red bell peppers, cherries, and—cunningly hidden by the green pigment chlorophyll—spinach leaves), astaxanthin (found in wild salmon and lobster), and lycopene (found in tomato, watermelon, beets, and grapefruit).

Chlorophyll

Oxygenates the blood and helps the body to detox. A green beauty hero found in cucumber, parsley, and all green leafy vegetables.

Flavonoids

Work as antioxidants and are thought to protect against inflammations and various diseases. Present in many enjoyable things, such as cacao, green tea, pomegranate, and red wine. The flavonoid family is huge—some of its more famous stars are gingerol (ginger), kaempferol (fennel, cauliflower, leek, tomato), and quercetin (yellow onion, raw apple, green tea).

Resveratrol

A type of polyphenol, which in plants triggers processes that put the cells in defensive mode when external threats approach. Present in the skin of red grapes and lingonberries.

PROBIOTICS AND PREBIOTICS

Question: What's most important for glowing skin—a superexpensive serum or a stable intestinal flora? Answer: A stable intestinal flora (many who have been ill or on antibiotics know the truth of this). Probiotics are good bacteria, of which we want plenty in our intestines. Naturally present in fermented foods, such as yogurt, kimchi, miso, and kombucha, and as a supplement. Prebiotics are types of fiber that feed the stomach's bacteria so that they can thrive and multiply. Present in several common vegetables, such as onions, artichoke, garlic, and beans, and in my favorite sweetener, yacon syrup. The skin's bacterial flora is a research topic on the rise, and we will certainly see more of it in probiotic skincare in the future.

VITAMINS

A bunch of organic substances that are necessary for our bodies, and which we can only obtain through food. Vitamins A, D, E, and K are fat-soluble and must be eaten with fat to be absorbed. Vitamins C and B are water soluble.

Index

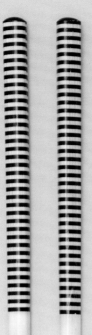

Further reading

EAT PRETTY: NUTRITION FOR BEAUTY, INSIDE AND OUT
Jolene Hart (Chronicle Books, San Francisco, 2014)

STORA BOKEN OM VITAMINER
Klaus Oberbeil (Wahlström & Widstrand, Stockholm, 2002)

FOREVER YOUNG: THE SCIENCE OF NUTRIGENOMICS FOR GLOWING, WRINKLE-FREE SKIN AND RADIANT HEALTH AT EVERY AGE
Nicholas Perricone (Atria Books, New York, 2010)

EAT BEAUTIFUL: FOOD AND RECIPES TO NOURISH YOUR SKIN FROM THE INSIDE OUT
Wendy Rowe (Clarkson Potter Publishers, New York, 2016)

THE BEAUTY DETOX SOLUTION: EAT YOUR WAY TO RADIANT SKIN, RENEWED ENERGY AND THE BODY YOU'VE ALWAYS WANTED
Kimberly Snyder (Harlequin Books, Toronto, 2011)

FEED YOUR FACE: YOUNGER, SMOOTHER SKIN AND A BEAUTIFUL BODY IN 28 DELICIOUS DAYS
Jessica Wu (St. Martin's Press, New York, 2011)

"DIET AND ACNE: A REVIEW OF THE EVIDENCE"
Elsa H. Spencer, Hope R. Ferdowsian and Neal D. Barnard (International Journal of Dermatology, no. 48, pp.339–47, 2009)

"KAROTENOIDER—KAROTENER OCH XANTOFYLLER SOM ANTIOXIDANTER" (CAROTENOIDS—CAROTENE AND XANTHOPHYLLS AS ANTIOXIDANTS
Göran Petersson (Chalmers Publication Library, Gothenburg, 2009)

Thanks

Lina, for your magical photos, and Helena, for your design genius. Making this book with two of my best friends was such a luxury. You're my superteam.

Cassandra Wikman, the dream production assistant, for exemplary insights ranging from mixers to face mist. You are my starlet 4-ever.

Michaéla Marmgren at Norstedts, because you believed in *Beauty Food* and in us. You made all this possible.

My publisher Gunilla and my editor Hedvig for your sharpness and knowledge.

Mia Högfeldt and Eva and Jennie at Forces for cheekbones and glow on D-day.

Damernas Värld editorial for making every day a party. You are world class.

Thanks to Greta for letting us use your dollhouse kitchen to shoot in.

Mom, because you always, through thick and thin, believe in me and support me.

Dad, my brothers, and my parents-in-law for enthusiasm and cheering me on.

Last, but not least, Vera and Christoffer. You are everything. I live with a chronically swollen heart thanks to you. ♡

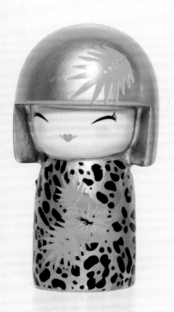
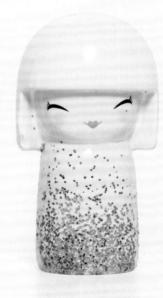
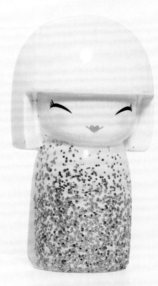

FOLLOW ME @MARIA_AHLGREN ON INSTAGRAM

An Hachette UK Company
www.hachette.co.uk

First published in Great Britain in 2018 by Mitchell Beazley,
an imprint of Octopus Publishing Group Ltd
Carmelite House
50 Victoria Embankment
London EC4Y 0DZ
www.octopusbooks.co.uk

First published as *Beauty Food* by Norstedts, Sweden in 2017

This edition published in the US in 2021 by agreement with
Norstedts Förlag

Distributed in the US by Hachette Book Group
1290 Avenue of the Americas
4th and 5th Floors
New York, NY 10104

Distributed in Canada by Canadian Manda Group
664 Annette St.Toronto, Ontario, Canada M6S 2C8

ISBN 978 1 78472 754 3

Printed and bound in China

10 9 8 7 6 5 4 3 2 1

All reasonable care has been taken in the preparation of this book
but the information it contains is not intended to take the place
of treatment or advice given by a qualified medical practitioner.

Before making any changes to your skincare routine, always
consult a specialist. While all the therapies detailed in this book
are completely safe if done correctly, you must seek professional
advice if you have any existing skin conditions or concerns. Any
application of the ideas and information contained in this book
are at the reader's sole discretion and risk.

Commissioning Editor: Joe Cottington
Editorial Assistant: Emily Brickell
Junior Designer: Jack Storey
Translator: Christian Gullette
Senior Production Controller: Allison Gonsalves
Photography: Lina Eidenberg Adamo
Design: Helena Radelius